[

CALCIUM NUTRITURE
FOR
MOTHERS AND CHILDREN

Carnation Nutrition Education Series

Calcium Nutriture
for
Mothers and Children

Editors

Reginald C. Tsang, M.B.B.S.

Gamble Professor of Neonatology
Executive Director, Perinatal Research
Institute
Children's Hospital
University of Cincinnati Medical Center
Cincinnati, Ohio

Francis Mimouni, M.D.

Associate Professor
Pediatrics, Obstetrics, and Gynecology
Magee-Womens Hospital
Pittsburgh, Pennsylvania

Carnation Nutrition
Education Series
Volume 3

CARNATION EDUCATION

RAVEN PRESS ■ NEW YORK

Carnation Co., 800 North Brand Boulevard, Glendale, California 91203
Raven Press, Ltd., 1185 Avenue of the Americas, New York, New York 10036

Made in the United States of America

Library of Congress Cataloging-in-Publication Data

Calcium nutriture for mothers and children / editors, Reginald C.
    Tsang, Francis Mimouni.
        p.   cm.—(Carnation nutrition education series ; v. 3)
    Based on a symposium held in Cincinnati, Nov. 1990.
    Includes index.
    ISBN 0-88167-869-4
    1. Pregnancy—Nutritional aspects—Congresses. 2. Children—
Nutrition—Congresses. 3. Calcium in human nutrition—Congresses.
I. Tsang, Reginald C. II. Mimouni, Francis. III. Series.
    [DNLM: 1. Bone and Bones—metabolism—congresses.
2. Calcium—metabolism—congresses. 3. Metabolism—in infancy &
childhood—congresses. 4. Metabolism—in pregnancy—congresses.
5. Vitamin D—physiology—congresses.   W1 CA835L v. 3 1990 /
QV 276 C1439   1990]
RG559.C33   1992
612.3'924—dc20
DNLM/DLC   91-35187
for Library of Congress   CIP

The material contained in this volume was submitted as previously unpublished material, except in the instances in which credit has been given to the source from which some of the illustrative material was derived.

Great care has been taken to maintain the accuracy of the information contained in the volume. However, neither Carnation nor Raven Press can be held responsible for errors or for any consequences arising from the use of the information contained herein.

9 8 7 6 5 4 3 2 1

Contents

Contributing Authors

Louis V. Avioli, M.D.
Director, Division of Bone and Mineral
  Diseases
Washington University School of Medicine
660 South Euclid Avenue
St. Louis, Missouri 63110
Chief, Section of Endocrinology and
  Metabolism
The Jewish Hospital of St. Louis
St. Louis, Missouri 63110

Russell W. Chesney, M.D.
Le Bonheur Professor and Chair
Department of Pediatrics
The University of Tennessee, Memphis
848 Adams Avenue, Suite 306
Memphis, Tennessee 38103
Vice President for Academic Affairs
Le Bonheur Children's Medical Center
Memphis, Tennessee 38103

Maria Lourdes A. Cruz, M.D.
Department of Pediatrics
The Division of Neonatology
The Perinatal Research Institute
University of Cincinnati College of Medicine
231 Bethesda Avenue
Cincinnati, Ohio 45267–0541

Frank R. Greer, M.D.
Professor, Department of Pediatrics
University of Wisconsin
600 Highland Avenue
Madison, Wisconsin 53706

Heidi J. Kalkwarf, Ph.D.
Research Fellow, Department of
  Neonatology
Children's Hospital Medical Center
Elland and Bethesda Avenues
Cincinnati, Ohio 45299–2899

Winston W.K. Koo, M.B.B.S.
Associate Professor
Departments of Pediatrics and Obstetrics and
  Gynecology
The University of Tennessee, Memphis
853 Jefferson Avenue
Memphis, Tennessee 38163

Francis Mimouni, M.D.
Associate Director
Departments of Pediatrics, Obstetrics, and
  Gynecology
Magee-Womens Hospital
University of Pittsburgh School of Medicine
Forbes Avenue and Halket Street
Pittsburgh, Pennsylvania 15213–3180

Leslie Myatt, Ph.D.
Associate Professor
Perinatal Research Institute
Department of Obstetrics and Gynecology,
  Pediatrics, and Physiology and Biophysics
University of Cincinnati College of Medicine
231 Bethesda Avenue
Cincinnati, Ohio, 45267–0526

Jay A. Perman, M.D.
Associate Professor
Department of Pediatrics
Division of Gastroenterology and Nutrition
Johns Hopkins University School of Medicine
600 North Wolfe Street
Baltimore, Maryland 21205

Roy M. Pitkin, M.D.
Professor and Chairman
Department of Obstetrics and Gynecology
University of California, Los Angeles, School
  of Medicine
10833 Le Conte Avenue, Room 27–117 CHS
Los Angeles, California 90024–1740

Bonny L. Specker, Ph.D.
Associate Professor
Department of Pediatrics
University of Cincinnati Medical Center
231 Bethesda Avenue
Cincinnati, Ohio 45267–0541

Reginald C. Tsang, M.B.B.S.
Executive Director
The Perinatal Research Institute
Department of Pediatrics
The Division of Neonatology
University of Cincinnati College of Medicine
231 Bethesda Avenue
Cincinnati, Ohio 45267–0541

Preface

Currently, there is a national concern and focus on osteoporosis. Millions of older Americans are afflicted with osteoporosis and its resultant propensity for fractures and disability. However, very little is known about the genesis of this disorder, and particularly if its origins can be traced to infancy and childhood. The present symposium is an exciting prelude to major advances in the decades to come, as scientists turn their attention to long-term bone health, starting from infancy (or even the fetus?).

Assembled together for a one day symposia in Cincinnati were some of the world's leading authorities on maternal, infant, and childhood calcium and bone metabolism. The speakers presented up-to-date information on bone health development to the assembled audience of pediatricians, obstetricians, nurses, dietitians, and allied health professionals.

This book summarizes the important information presented that day. Dr. Reginald Tsang begins by presenting the basics of mineral metabolism, and by establishing the breast fed infant as the "gold standard." Dr. Roy Pitkin discusses the pregnant and lactating female, including the impact of diet and teen pregnancy on pregnancy outcome and lactation. Dr. Francis Mimouni examines vitamin D requirements in the first year of life, particularly as it relates to season, culture, and racial factors. Dr. Frank Greer explores calcium needs and metabolism during childhood and adolescence, focusing on the impact of calcium intake. Dr. Louis Avioli investigates the potential relationship of childhood bone development to osteoporosis in adulthood. Dr. Jay Perman assesses the potential impact of lactose intolerance and diets without lactose in calcium metabolism.

This book also discusses important clinical issues. Dr. Bonny Specker explores mineral and vitamin D requirements in lactation. Dr. Russell Chesney discusses the assessment of bone mineral status and dietary mineral adequacy, and new techniques of measurement of bone mineral content. Dr. Winston Koo deals with meeting calcium needs in the premature infant through parenteral and enteral nutrition. Dr. Leslie Myatt examines the relationship of mineral nutrition and metabolism to preeclampsia and premature labor, also emphasizing potential adverse effects of high-dose calcium.

This volume of presentations by experts in the field of maternal-fetal, infant, and juvenile mineral metabolism allows a unique glimpse at the potential impact of early childhood bone development on subsequent bone health. We hope the reader will be stimulated to read further on the subject, utilizing the many references in the present volume, and to stay tuned to this exciting developing field.

REGINALD C. TSANG, M.B.B.S.
FRANCIS MIMOUNI, M.D.

Acknowledgments

The editors would like to acknowledge the help of Russell Merritt, M.D., Ph.D., Medical and Scientific Director; Linda Hsieh, R.D., Assistant Manager, Medical Education, Carnation Nutrition Product Division; Pam Weiss, Manager, Scientific Services; and John P. White, R.Ph., Vice President, Scientific Services, M.E.D. Communications, for their efforts in arranging for publication of this book. The editors also wish to thank the organizers of the Symposium Bare Bones Nutrition, *Current Clinical Perspectives on Calcium in Pregnancy, Infancy, and Childhood,* Jill Kriser and Charlotte VanDuser, Account Executives, Bill Com Exposition and Conference Group, and Donna Buckley, Perinatal Research Institute, Children's Hospital and University of Cincinnati, for their efficient organization of the symposium.

Calcium Nutriture for Mothers and Children, edited by Reginald C. Tsang and Francis Mimouni. Carnation Nutrition Education Series, Vol. 3. Carnation Co., Glendale/Raven Press, Ltd., New York © 1992.

Introduction to Infant Mineral Metabolism

Maria Lourdes A. Cruz and Reginald C. Tsang

Department of Pediatrics, The Division of Neonatology, The Perinatal Research Institute, University of Cincinnati College of Medicine, Cincinnati, Ohio 45267-0541

Calcium (Ca) and phosphorus (P) metabolism are intimately related, and both minerals arc closcly related to vitamin D, parathyroid (PTH), and calcitonin (CT) metabolism. Infant mineral metabolism involves major additional variables including development, growth, and diet. In the present introduction, we will concentrate on infants fed the gold standard for infant diet, human milk, to develop the concept of *normal physiology*.

CALCIUM

Calcium is the most abundant mineral in the body. Serum Ca concentration is tightly regulated and is dependent on the interplay of various hormones on the intestine, bone, and kidney to maintain the Ca pool (1) (Fig. 1). Briefly, PTH increases serum Ca concentrations by mobilizing Ca from bone, increasing renal tubular Ca reabsorption, and stimulating renal 1,25 dihydroxyvitamin D [$1,25(OH)_2D$] production. $1,25(OH)_2D$ increases intestinal Ca absorption, renal Ca reabsorption, and mobilization of Ca from bone. CT lowers serum Ca concentrations by inhibiting bone resorption and possibly increasing renal Ca clearance. PTH and CT are subject to feedback regulation by serum Ca concentrations: high serum Ca concentrations inhibit PTH secretion but stimulate CT production. In addition, Ca and P metabolism are closely linked so that serum concentrations of one mineral affect serum concentrations of the other mineral. These regulatory mechanisms are functional in the normal full-term infant. The role of diet as an important determinant of the type and magnitude of these responses will be highlighted in the following discussion.

The absorption of Ca apparently occurs by both active and passive mechanisms throughout the small intestine, primarily in the duodenum (2). The bioavailability of Ca in human milk is high, so that the percentage of Ca absorbed is higher for human milk compared with cow milk-derived formulas. However, the absolute quantity of Ca absorbed from human milk is lower because of its lower Ca content (approximately 40 versus 56–75 mg/100 kcal in cow milk-derived formulas) (3). Bone mineral content (BMC), a practical end point for Ca absorption and retention, may be similar among human milk- and formula-fed infants, or it may be lower in human milk-fed

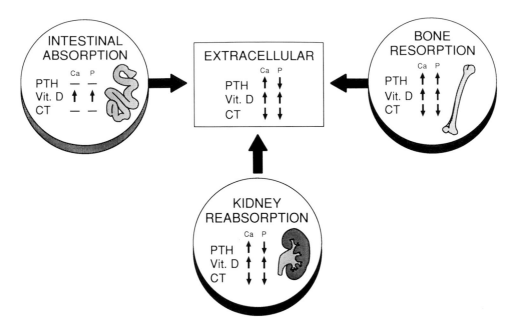

FIG. 1. Effects of various calciotropic hormones on different organ systems and their overall effects on serum calcium (*Ca*) and phosphorus (*P*) concentrations. Parathyroid hormone (*PTH*) increases bone release of Ca and P, and increases renal Ca reabsorption and P excretion, resulting in an overall increase in serum Ca but decrease in P concentrations. Vitamin D (*Vit. D*), like 1,25,(OH)$_2$D, stimulates intestinal Ca and P absorption, bone Ca and P resorption, and renal Ca and P reabsorption, resulting in an overall increase in serum Ca and P concentrations. Calcitonin (*CT*) acts mainly to decrease bone resorption and renal reabsorption of Ca and P, resulting in an overall decrease in serum Ca and P concentrations.

infants (Fig. 2) (4). Other factors that theoretically increase Ca absorption include the presence of lactose, medium-chain triglycerides (1), and high intraluminal concentrations of Ca and P (2).

Whether Ca absorption in the neonatal period is vitamin D-dependent remains controversial; some investigators have suggested that Ca absorption is linear with intake and is not vitamin D dependent, whereas others have presented evidence that Ca absorption is vitamin D dependent (5–7). For example, one study demonstrated an increase in Ca absorption from a value of 50 percent in preterm infants fed human milk not supplemented with vitamin D, compared with a value of 74 percent in matched infants fed vitamin D- and P-supplemented human milk (7). Ca retentions were 31–34% compared with 64%, respectively.

Ca loss occurs primarily via the fecal route; part of the loss is related to endogenous intestinal secretory losses ranging from 1 percent to 50 percent of the calcium intake (5). Urinary losses, which are normally low in infancy, can also occur secondary to increased sodium, protein, and glucose intake (2).

The Ca to P ratio (Ca:P) and the adequacy of P in the diet play important roles

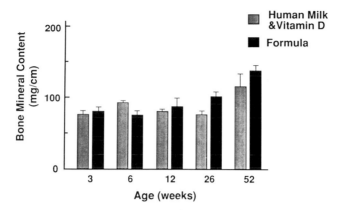

FIG. 2. Bone mineral content in term infants as affected by diet. Age of infants in weeks is plotted on the *x* axis. Bone mineral content in mg/cm is plotted on the *y* axis. Infants on human milk with vitamin D supplements are represented by the hatched bars. There was a progressive increase in bone mineral content in both groups over the first year of life, with no significant difference between the two groups from 3 to 52 weeks of age. (Data derived from Greer and McCormick, ref. 14, with permission.)

in the retention of these minerals. A Ca:P ratio of roughly 2:1 in the diet, the ratio found in human milk, appears to be optimal for term infants. Currently, because of the inherent high P content and low Ca:P ratio of cow milk, and due to technical difficulties in decreasing P content, most proprietary cow milk-derived infant formulas have a higher P content and lower Ca:P ratio (1.3:1) compared with human milk.

The differences in Ca and P contents between human and cow milk are reflected in the serum concentrations of these minerals in the infants receiving these two different milk types. In the first 6 months of life and with increasing age, serum P concentrations fall, and serum Ca concentrations rise, in human milk-fed term infants (Fig. 3) (8). Because of their higher dietary phosphate load, cow milk-derived formula-fed term infants have higher serum P and lower ionized Ca concentrations compared with human milk-fed infants (Fig. 4) (9). The lowered ionized Ca concentrations may cause some formula-fed infants to develop "late onset" neonatal tetany.

No major deficiency of Ca or P intake has been demonstrated in healthy term infants fed human milk. The Ca requirement in term infants fed cow milk-derived formula is approximately 60 mg/kg/day (2).

In growing preterm infants fed human milk, the Ca and especially P contents in human milk are low relative to their rapid growth needs during this period. Low P intake in preterm infants fed human milk may lead to significant hypophosphatemia, which leads to hypercalcemia and secondary hypercalciuria. The calcium losses aggravate the already calcium-deficient state, relative to intrauterine mineral needs, and bone mineralization is compromised. Osteopenia or rickets may then ensue (10,11). Supplemental Ca and P may be of benefit in these infants. Several studies

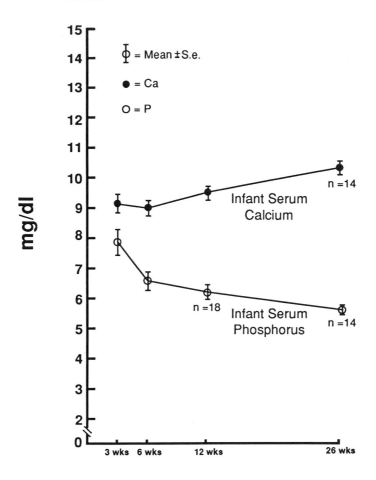

Age in Weeks

FIG. 3. Serum Ca and P over time in human milk-fed infants followed in a longitudinal study. The age of infants in weeks after birth is plotted on the x axis. Serum mineral concentrations in mg/dl are plotted on the y axis. Closed circles represent serum calcium (Ca) concentrations; open circles represent serum phosphorus (P) concentrations. There is a progressive increase in serum Ca concentrations ($p < 0.005$), and a decrease in serum P concentrations in human milk fed infants in the first 6 months of life ($p < 0.001$). (Adapted from Greer et al., *J Pediatr* 1982;100:59–64, with permission.)

have evaluated the efficacy of human milk fortifiers for the prevention of osteopenia in human milk-fed preterm infants (12–14). BMC is improved in preterm infants fed protein- and mineral-fortified human milk compared with preterm infants fed unfortified human milk, and is comparable to BMCs of infants receiving proprietary fortified preterm milk formula (13). Absorption of the supplemental Ca is similar to absorption of endogenously labeled Ca in human milk (i.e., stable isotopes given to

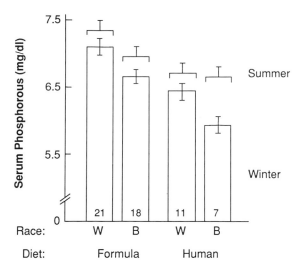

FIG. 4. Serum P concentrations in infants less than 6 months by race, diet, and season. The variables race [white (W) versus black (B)] and diet (formula versus human milk) are plotted on the *x* axis. Serum phosphorus concentration in mg/dl is plotted on the *y* axis. The lower bars represent measurements taken in winter; the upper bars represent measurements taken in summer. Numbers within the bars are numbers of infants studied. Black infants had a significantly lower serum P concentration compared with white infants ($p < 0.001$). Formula-fed infants had significantly higher serum P concentrations compared with human milk-fed infants ($p < 0.001$). Serum P concentrations were significantly lower in winter than in summer ($p < 0.001$). (Adapted from Specker et al., ref. 8, with permission.)

lactating women, appearing in milk) (15). In our nursery, Ca and P supplementation with either powdered fortifier (Enfamil, 1 packet/50 cc of human milk) or liquid fortifiers (Similac Natural Care, 1:1 mix) is recommended for growing preterm infants when intake of human milk reaches 130–150 ml/kg/day; infants are gradually weaned from the fortifier before discharge (16). Preterm infants fed cow milk-derived formulas may have Ca requirements up to 200 mg/kg/day (2).

PHOSPHORUS

Phosphorus, along with Ca, is essential for bone mineralization. Serum P concentrations are regulated by the same hormones that control serum Ca concentrations (1) (Fig. 1). PTH and CT increase renal P excretion; CT antagonizes the resorptive action of PTH on bone. Together, these effects result in reduced serum P concentrations. 1,25(OH)$_2$D increases intestinal P absorption, thereby increasing serum P concentrations.

Intestinal absorption of P is very high in infancy, apparently occurring throughout the small intestine (2). As with Ca, P is probably absorbed by both passive and active mechanisms. In contrast to Ca, 80–90 percent of P intake is absorbed and retained.

In spite of the extremely high fractional absorption and retention of P, however, the low P content of human milk [19 mg/100 kcal in human milk compared with 42–58 mg/100 kcal in cow milk-derived formula (3)] results in low net absorption and retention of P in preterm infants.

Urinary P excretion in the neonate is acutely sensitive to dietary P intake. P deprivation in infants rapidly results in marked reduction in urinary P excretion. Infants who are fed human milk, especially those who are preterm, have an extremely low P excretion as a response to the low P content of human milk (2). This finding probably reflects an efficient renal P conservation mechanism at a time of maximal P need and utilization. However, in spite of this efficient conservation mechanism, significant hypophosphatemia may occur in preterm infants receiving human milk. Low dietary P intake and high P needs for bone mineralization predispose preterm infants toward the development of rickets (17).

As mentioned earlier, serum P concentrations are higher in cow milk-derived formula-fed infants compared with human milk-fed infants. Factors other than diet that may affect serum P concentrations are race and season; serum P concentrations are lower in black infants compared with white infants and in winter compared with summer (Fig. 4) (8). The reasons for the race and seasonal differences are unclear, but might be related to vitamin D physiology (see below).

Human milk-fed term infants receive sufficient P to meet their requirements. The daily enteric requirement for P is approximately 40 mg/kg/day in term infants fed cow milk-derived formulas (2). For reasons explained earlier, the preterm infant who has not had the benefit of maximal intrauterine P accretion and who is fed exclusively with human milk probably needs P and Ca supplementation. In preterm infants fed cow milk-derived formula, the P requirements may reach 100–120 mg/kg/day (2).

VITAMIN D

Vitamin D plays an integral part in Ca metabolism and is mainly supplied by two routes: oral intake as exogenous vitamin D_2 and D_3 mostly from vitamin D-fortified milk and milk products (in certain countries including the United States), and endogenous production by the skin (Fig. 5). Vitamin D production by the skin occurs through the conversion of provitamin D_3 to previtamin D_3 under ultraviolet B radiation; previtamin D_3 is then converted into vitamin D_3. Hydroxylation of both exogenous and endogenous vitamin D_2 and D_3 to 25-hydroxyvitamin D (25-OHD) then takes place in the liver. Most workers consider the serum concentration of total 25-OHD to be an index of vitamin D status, with low concentrations indicative of inadequate vitamin D stores. 25-OHD is further converted into the active metabolite $1,25(OH)_2D$ in the kidney (3). $1,25(OH)_2D$ increases intestinal Ca and P absorption, mobilizes Ca and P from bone, and facilitates renal Ca and P reabsorption. Its blood concentrations are elevated in the presence of low Ca or P intake, or during periods of increased Ca and P needs. Low serum Ca concentrations stimulate production of PTH, which in turn results in elevation of $1,25(OH)_2D$ concentrations. Low serum

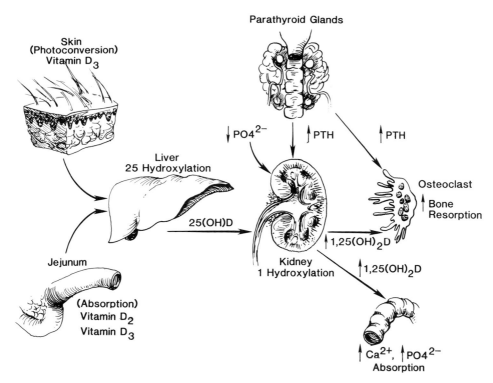

FIG. 5. Normal vitamin D metabolism. Vitamin D_2 from diet, and vitamin D_3 from diet and skin photoconversion, are hydroxylated in the liver to 25-OHD. 25-OHD undergoes further hydroxylation in the kidney to form 1,25,(OH)$_2$D, which is stimulated by parathyroid hormone (PTH). 1,25(OH)$_2$D is responsible for increasing bone resorption and intestinal calcium and phosphorus absorption. PTH acts synergistically with 1,25(OH)$_2$D to increase bone resorption.

P concentrations are also a potent stimulus for 1,25(OH)$_2$D production. Thus, the serum 1,25(OH$_2$)D concentration is an excellent index of Ca and P status.

The vitamin D status at birth depends on maternal vitamin D status (18). Infant cord blood 25-OHD concentrations correlate directly with maternal serum concentrations (19). After birth, the vitamin D status of infants depends on vitamin D exogenously derived from milk intake and endogenously synthesized from sunshine exposure. Serum 25-OHD concentrations in exclusively breast-fed infants may (20) or may not (21) correlate with vitamin D content of human milk. Vitamin D content of human milk, in turn, correlates directly with maternal intake of vitamin D, and increases acutely with daily maternal vitamin D supplementation (2,000 IU) for 2 weeks (22). Judged by plasma 25-OHD concentrations, the vitamin D stores of most breast-fed infants born to mothers with normal vitamin D status are depleted approximately 8 weeks after delivery (Fig. 6) (23). Since vitamin D concentrations in human milk are normally much lower than in commercial milk formulas [3 IU/100 kcal in human milk versus 60–62 IU/100 kcal in cow milk-derived vitamin D-fortified

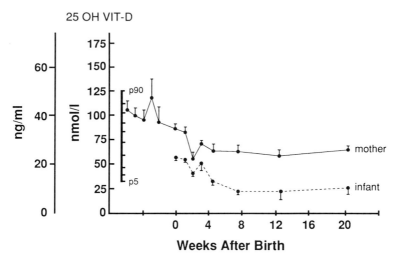

FIG. 6. Serum vitamin D concentrations in human milk-fed infants not receiving vitamin D supplements over time. Age of infants in weeks is plotted on the x axis. Serum 25-OHD concentrations in nmol/l (and in ng/ml) are plotted on the y axis. The fifth (*p5*) and ninetieth percentiles (*p90*) for normal serum 25-OHD concentrations, calculated using the bootstrap technique, are indicated on the left. Maternal serum 25-OHD concentrations are represented by the solid lines. Infant serum 25-OHD concentrations are represented by the dotted lines. There was a progressive decline in serum 25-OHD concentrations in both mother and infant over time. Infant serum 25-OHD concentrations were significantly lower than the fifth percentile by age 8 weeks. (Adapted from Hoogenboezem et al., ref. 23, with permission.)

formulas (2)], it is not surprising that serum 25-OHD concentrations in human milk-fed infants are lower than in formula-fed infants (Fig. 7) (22). Thus, even the term infant who is exclusively breastfed theoretically might be at risk for vitamin D deficiency unless there is adequate sunshine exposure.

There may be adaptive mechanisms in infants in response to vitamin D status. In a study by Lichtenstein et al. in Cincinnati (24), the serum concentration of $1,25(OH)_2D$ at 0–18 months of age was higher in black versus white infants and in infants in winter versus those in summer (Fig. 8). At 6 days of age, serum $1,25(OH)_2D$ concentrations may also be higher in human milk-fed infants compared with vitamin D-fortified formula-fed infants (25). These findings lead us to speculate that infants may have the ability to respond to situations of decreased vitamin D supply (because of dark pigmentation, and/or decreased sunshine exposure during the winter season, or low dietary vitamin D) by increasing production of the active metabolite $1,25(OH)_2D$. Since low serum P concentrations are also seen in black and human milk-fed infants, and during winter (Fig. 4), we suggest that low serum 25-OHD concentrations result in low serum P concentrations, which in turn result in increased $1,25(OH)_2D$ concentrations in order to maintain overall P economy.

There have been some reports of rickets in term infants exclusively receiving human milk (26,27). In these infants, however, deficiency of vitamin D appears to be related either to inadequate sunshine exposure or probable maternal vitamin D

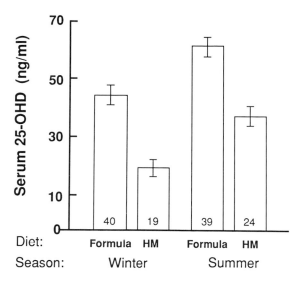

FIG. 7. Serum 25-OHD concentrations as affected by diet and season. The variables diet [formula versus human milk (*HM*)] and season (winter versus summer) are plotted on the x axis. Numbers within the bars are numbers of infants studied. Serum 25(OH)D concentrations in ng/ml are plotted on the Y axis. Serum 25-OHD concentrations were significantly lower in human milk-fed infants ($p < 0.001$) and during winter ($p < 0.001$). (From Lichtenstein et al., ref. 24, with permission.)

deficiency or osteomalacia. In northern latitudes, where daylight exposure is markedly diminished, infants who are exclusively breastfed have serum 25-OHD concentrations in the rachitic range (28). Saudi Arabian infants nursed by mothers with very little sunshine exposure because of traditional dress habits and inadequate dietary vitamin D show low serum 25-OHD concentrations (29). Thus, although human milk is generally considered the standard in reference to early infant nutrient requirements, it should not be considered as an adequate source of vitamin D in conditions of low sunshine exposure or low maternal vitamin D status.

The vitamin D status of human milk-fed infants may be increased either by increasing sunshine exposure or directly supplementing the infants with 400 IU of vitamin D daily. Increasing sunshine exposure increases serum 25-OHD concentrations in exclusively breast-fed babies (30). In term infants, very minimal sunshine exposure [10–30 minutes of hand and face exposure per week (31)], may result in normal serum vitamin D concentrations. Thus, no further vitamin D supplementation in these situations appears to be necessary. However, there may be a role for vitamin D supplementation in exclusively breast-fed infants living in extremely northern latitudes, particularly if they are dark skinned, living in circumstances that restrict sun exposure, or born during prolonged winter seasons, or in infants whose mothers are vitamin D deficient due to either diet or dress customs.

It may also be prudent to supplement vitamin D in preterm infants fed human milk. Although the major problem leading to osteopenia and rickets in these infants is Ca and P mineral deficiency (32), this problem theoretically might be exacerbated

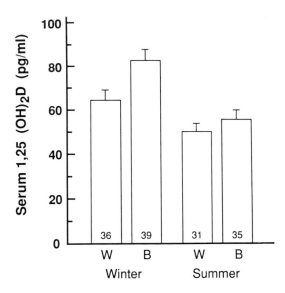

FIG. 8. Serum 1,25(OH)$_2$D concentrations as affected by race and season. The variables race [white (*W*) versus black (*B*)] and season (winter versus summer) are plotted on the *x* axis. Serum 1,25(OH)$_2$D concentrations (in pg/ml) are plotted on the *y* axis. Numbers within the bars are numbers of infants studied. Serum 1,25(OH)$_2$D concentrations were significantly higher in black infants ($p < 0.001$) and during winter ($p < 0.001$). (From Lichtenstein et al., ref. 24, with permission.)

by the usual lack of sun exposure in the nursery and the usually low vitamin D content of human milk. Approximately 400 IU of vitamin D per day for these infants is probably sufficient. Higher doses do not appear to be necessary and have not been shown to prevent or successfully treat the bone disturbance.

In summary, the metabolism of Ca, P, and vitamin D in infancy is influenced by the type of nutrition that the infant receives. Human milk remains the norm for nutrition for the term infant in regard to Ca and P metabolism. The intestinal fractional absorption of Ca and P from human milk is high in term infants. The vitamin D content of human milk correlates directly with maternal vitamin D intake and status. In certain situations it may be prudent to add vitamin D to the diet of exclusively breast-fed term infants, such as those who receive inadequate sun exposure or whose mothers are vitamin D deficient. Otherwise, in general, human milk maintains adequate Ca, P, and vitamin D status in term, healthy white infants. However, in preterm infants, the Ca and P content of human milk is low relative to mineral needs; hypophosphatemia is common in these infants. It may be judicious to supplement growing preterm infants exclusively fed human milk with Ca and P fortifiers as well as 400 IU daily of vitamin D.

ACKNOWLEDGMENTS

This work was supported in part by NIH grant HD 11725, USPHS Training in Perinatal Care and Research grant MCH MCT 000174, NIH Clinical Research Center grant RR00068, NIH grant 20748, and the Perinatal Research Institute.

REFERENCES

1. Koo WWK, Tsang RC. Calcium and magnesium in health and disease. In: Werner M, ed. *Clinical research center handbook of clinical chemistry,* vol 4. Orlando: CRC Press, 1989;51–91.
2. Koo WWK, Tsang RC. Calcium, magnesium, and phosphorus. In: Tsang RC, Nichols BL, eds. *Nutrition during infancy.* Philadelphia: Hanley & Belfus, 1988;175–189.
3. Tsang RC, Nichols BL, ed. *Nutrition during infancy.* Philadelphia: Hanley & Belfus, 1988;419 (Appendix).
4. Barltrop D, Mole R, Sutton A. Absorption and endogenous fecal excretion of calcium by low birth weight infants on feeds with varying contents of calcium and phosphate. *Arch Dis Child* 1977;52:41–49.
5. Senterre J, Putet G, Salle B, et al. Effects of vitamin D and phosphorus supplementation on calcium retention in preterm infants fed banked human milk. *J Pediatr* 1983;103:305–307.
6. Senterre J, Salle B. Calcium and phosphorus economy of the preterm infant and its interaction with vitamin D and its metabolites. *Acta Paediatr Scand [Suppl]* 1982;296:85–92.
7. Greer FR, Tsang RC, Levin RS, Searcy JE, Wu R, Steichen JJ. Increasing serum calcium and magnesium concentrations in breast-fed infants: longitudinal studies of minerals in human milk and in sera of nursing mothers and their infants. *J Pediatr* 1982;100:59–64.
8. Specker BL, Lichtenstein P, Mimouni F, Gormley C, Tsang RC. Calcium-regulating hormones and minerals from birth to 18 months of age: a cross-sectional study. II. Effects of sex, race, age, season, and diet on serum minerals, parathyroid hormone, and calcitonin. *Pediatrics* 1986;77:891–896.
9. Greer FR, Searcy JE, Levin RS, Steichen JJ, Asch PS, Tsang RC. Bone mineral content and serum 15-hydroxyvitamin D concentration in breastfed infants with and without supplemental vitamin D. *J Pediatr* 1981;98:696–701.
10. Kulkarni PB, Hall RT, Rhodes PG, et al. Rickets in very low birth weight infants. *J Pediatr* 1980;96:249–252.
11. Halbert KE, Tsang RC. Rickets in the newborn period and premature infants. In: Castells S, Finberg L, eds. *Metabolic bone disease in children.* New York: Marcel Dekker, Inc., 1990;99–150.
12. Greer FR, Steichen JJ, Tsang RC. Calcium and phosphate supplements in breast milk-related rickets. Results in a very-low-birth-weight infant. *Am J Dis Child* 1982;136:581–583.
13. Abrams SA, Schanler RJ, Garza C. Bone mineralization in former very low birth weight infants fed either human milk or commercial formula. *J Pediatr* 1988;112:956–960.
14. Greer FR, McCormick A. Improved bone mineralization and growth in premature infants fed fortified own mother's milk. *J Pediatr* 1988;112:961–969.
15. Liu YM, Neal P, Ernst J, et al. Absorption of calcium and magnesium from fortified human milk by very low birth weight infants. *Pediatr Res* 1989;25:496–502.
16. Niedbala BJ, Tsang RC. The small for gestational age infant. In: Ekvall S, ed. *Pediatric nutrition in chronic and developmental diseases.* Springfield, IL: Charles C Thomas, [In press].
17. Rowe J, Rowe D, Hovak E, et al. Hypophosphatemia and hypercalciuria in small premature infants fed human milk: evidence for inadequate dietary phosphorus. *J Pediatr* 1984;104:112–117.
18. Delvin EE, Glorieux FH, Salle BL, David L, Varenne JP. Control of vitamin D metabolism in preterm infants. Feto-maternal relationships. *Arch Dis Child* 1982;57:754–757.
19. Anderson DM, Hollis BW, LeVine BR, Pittard WB. Dietary assessment of maternal vitamin D intake and correlation with maternal and neonatal serum vitamin D concentrations at delivery. *J Perinatol* 1988;8:46–48.
20. Cancela L, Le Boulch N, Miravet L. Relationship between the vitamin D content of maternal milk and the vitamin D status of nursing women and breast-fed infants. *J Endocrinol* 1986;110:43–50.
21. Specker BL, Tsang RC, Hollis BW. Effect of race and diet on human milk vitamin D and 25-hydroxyvitamin D. *Am J Dis Child* 1985;139:1134–1137.
22. Hollis BW, Greer FR, Tsang RC. The effect of oral vitamin D supplementation and ultraviolet therapy on the antirachitic sterol content of human milk. *Tissue Int* 1982;34:552.
23. Hoogenboezem T, Degenhart HJ, de Muinck Keizer-Schrma SMPF DM, et al. Vitamin D metabolism in breast-fed infants and their mothers. *Pediatr Res* 1989;25:623–628.
24. Lichtenstein P, Specker BL, Tsang RC, Mimouni F, Gormley C. Calcium-regulating hormones and minerals from birth to 18 months of age: a cross sectional study. I. Effects of sex, race, age, season, and diet on vitamin D status. *Pediatrics* 1986;77:883–890.
25. Specker BL, Tsang RC, Ho ML, Landi TM, Gratton TL. Low serum calcium and high PTH in infants fed "humanized" cow milk based formula. *Am J Dis Child* 1991;145:941–945.

26. Edidin D, Levitsky LL, Schey W, Dumbovic N, Campos A. Resurgence of nutritional rickets associated with breastfeeding and special dietary practices. *Pediatrics* 1980;65:232–235.
27. Hayward I, Stein M, Gibson M. Nutritional rickets in San Diego. *Am J Dis Child* 1987;14:1060–1062.
28. Markestad T, Kolmannskog S, Arntzen E, Toftegaard L, Haneberg B, Aksnes L. Serum concentrations of vitamin D metabolites in exclusively breast-fed infants at 70 degrees North. *Acta Paediatr Scand* 1984;73:29–32.
29. Belton NR, Elidrissy ATH, Gaafer TH, et al. Maternal vitamin D deficiency as a factor in the pathogenesis of rickets in Saudi Arabia. In: Norman AW, Schaefer K, Herrath DV, Grigoleit HG, eds. *Vitamin D. Chemical, biochemical, and clinical endocrinology of calcium metabolism.* Berlin: de Gruyter, 1982;735–737.
30. Specker BL, Valanis B, Hertzberg V, Edwards N, Tsang RC. Sunshine exposure and serum 25-hydroxyvitamin D concentrations in exclusively breastfed infants. *J Pediatr* 1985;107:372–376.
31. Ho ML, Yen HC, Tsang RC, Specker BL, Chen XC, Nichols BL. Randomized study of sunshine exposure and serum 25-OHD in breastfed infants in Beijing, China. *J Pediatr* 1985;107:928–931.
32. Koo WWK, Sherman R, Succop P, Ho M, Buckley D, Tsang RC. Serum vitamin D metabolites in very low birth weight infants with and without rickets and fractures. *J Pediatr* 1989;114:1017–1022.

Calcium Nutriture for Mothers and Children, edited by
Reginald C. Tsang and Francis Mimouni. Carnation
Nutrition Education Series, Vol. 3. Carnation Co.,
Glendale/Raven Press, Ltd., New York © 1992.

Pediatric Calcium Needs and Metabolism Beyond Infancy

Frank R. Greer

Department of Pediatrics, University of Wisconsin, Madison 53706

The gold standard for calcium requirements in the first year of life is that determined from studies of breast-feeding infants, whether using metabolic balance techniques or measures of bone mineral content. For the period beyond infancy including adolescence, we have no comparable gold standard for determining pediatric calcium needs, and the exact requirements remain controversial. Dietary calcium intakes in children vary widely without obvious clinical signs of deficiency or excess. The body of the full-term newborn infant contains 25–30 g of calcium. The normal young adult contains 1,000–1,200 g of calcium, resulting in a net retention of about 1 kg of Ca between infancy and adulthood (1). The yearly net estimate for calcium retention varies with age (Table 1), with some relatively minor sex and ethnic differences.

The tenth edition of the Recommended Dietary Allowance (RDA) states that the calcium intake for children between the ages of 1 and 10 years should be at least 800 mg/day, though this allowance is thought to be arbitrary since specific data on requirements of this age group is lacking (2). These allowances are higher than those recommended by the World Health Organization (400–500 mg/day of calcium) for the same age group (3). As seen in Table 1, skeletal growth in these children requires at most 190 mg/day, so an intake of 800 mg/day would be very adequate. For adolescents, an RDA of 1,200 mg/day of calcium is recommended, the increase being necessary for the calcium requirements of the prepubertal growth spurt (net retention of 275–500 mg/day) (2). Again, the RDA is considerably higher than the World Health Organization's recommendation of 600–700 mg/day for adolescents (3).

As 99% of total body calcium is contained in the skeleton, one can argue that the primary pediatric calcium need is to support skeletal growth and maturation, which consists of three major phenomena:

1. Growth of the skeleton in length, volume and weight
2. Skeletal maturation or modeling, which includes consolidation of bone into its definitive form by enchondral ossification and the appearance of epiphyseal centers
3. Continuous remodeling and repair of bone tissue

The first and second phenomena occur only in children and adolescents. Growth

13

TABLE 1. *Net calcium retention with age*

Age (years)	Amount (grams per year)	Amount (mg/day)	Total[a] (grams)
0–2	70	190	140
2–8	20–25	55–68	120–150
8–10	50	137	100
10–18	80–100	219–274	640–800
Total			1,000–1,190

[a] Age (yr) × amount (g/yr) = total g.
Data from refs. 2 and 3.

ceases when the epiphyseal plates of long bones close (4). Skeletal maturation ends during adolescence when the bones have reached their final adult configuration, although some increase in bone mineral content continues through the third decade. The third phenomena persists throughout both childhood and adulthood.

The rigid nature of bone makes the interstitial growth characteristic of other tissues impossible. Increases in the size of the bone can only occur by the deposition of new tissue on the surfaces of preexisting bone. The growth of individual tubular bones is thus highly complex, as noted in the general description by Stanley Garn:

> The two ends of the bone grow at different yet changing rates, and the fast growing end at one age may be the slow growing end at another age. At one instant in time there may be rapid subperiosteal apposition near the elongating ends, rapid subperiosteal resorption some centimeters nearer the middle of the shaft, and slow subperiosteal apposition along the midshaft region (5).

Along with bone growth, bone modeling is also occurring in the child, in which bone formed at the wide epiphyseal plate is shaped to fit the thinner shaft by simultaneous bone resorption at the epiphyseal surface by osteoclasts and bone formation by osteoblasts at the endosteal surface. It took many years of observation to discern the peculiarities of bone growth. One of the initial important observations was made in 1736 by John Belchier, a surgeon. Dr. Belchier observed at the dinner table that the bones of pigs that had been fed on madder (the root of a Eurasian herb used for making dye) were colored red. Subsequently Duhamel, a French country squire, related the observation of madder staining to the mechanism of bone growth. In a series of experiments carried out between 1739 and 1743 he showed that madder colored those parts of the skeleton that were being formed at the time of its administration. Bone formed after withdrawing madder from the pig's diet was normally colored, and in certain regions this newly formed bone covered over the older bone, which retained its red discoloration. When madder feeding had been suspended for some weeks before the animal was killed, the ends of the shafts of long bone were found to be uncolored, suggesting end apposition was the mechanism for increasing bone length. From the layer of white bone ensheathing the midshaft region, Duhamel

TABLE 2. *Skeletal growth in the fetus, child, and adolescent*

Stage	Growth (cm)
Fetus	45–50
1st year	20
2nd year	10
3–12 years	5 cm/year
13–18 years	10 cm/year
Total	185

Data from Royer, ref. 1, and Sissons, ref. 4.

correctly inferred that a long bone grew in thickness, as did a tree, by the progressive development of new bone on its outer surface (4).

Skeletal growth varies with age, occurring at an approximate rate of 20–25 cm in the first year, 10 cm the second year, and 5 cm/year until the prepubertal period. Growth occurs at 10 cm/annum during the prepubertal years ceasing entirely about 4 years after the end of puberty (Table 2). Skeletal growth is also not homogeneous for different body segments. In girls, the highest rate of growth in the lower part of the body occurs before puberty, whereas the pubertal growth spurt occurs almost solely in the upper part of the body (1).

The exact mechanisms for the mineralization of growing bone are not clearly defined. Though the amount of bone mineral content (BMC) (so-called bone density) can be determined by a number of methods, single-photon absorptiometry has been most widely used in children. From 12 months to 6 years of age, BMC increases at a rate of 14%/year (6). Between the ages of 6 and 14 years, BMC increases at a rate of 10.5% annually (7,8). It is during adolescence that the most rapid weight gain of the skeleton occurs (Table 3). Although BMC may continue to increase well into the third decade of life, more significant increases in BMC occur during adolescence. The greatest increase in BMC occurs after the adolescent growth spurt has slowed

TABLE 3. *Radial bone mineral content (BMC) in infants, children, adolescents, and adults*

Stage	BMC (g/cm)
Birth	.090
6 years	.350–.460
14 years	.800–.900
20 years	.950–1.00
60 years	.770–1.226

Data from Specker et al., ref. 6, Mazess and Cameron, refs. 7, 8, and Krabbe et al., refs. 9, 10.

(9,10). This becomes significant as women who fail to generate their full adolescent bone mineral complement are more likely to develop symptomatic osteoporosis at an early age (11). There are sex differences in BMC; for example, the BMC of the radius is about 8% larger in boys than in girls from 6 to 13 years of age (12). There are also race differences; black adolescent females have a higher BMC than white adolescent females (13).

Numerous factors influence pediatric calcium needs and metabolism. These can be divided into three broad categories: (1) genetic and environmental factors; (2) hormonal factors (parathyroid hormone, vitamin D, calcitonin, growth hormones, thyroxine, sex hormones); and (3) factors affecting calcium availability and conservation (intestinal absorption, renal retention, nutritional status).

GENETIC AND ENVIRONMENTAL FACTORS

The ultimate needs for calcium to support growth are determined by genetic factors. Not only do genetic factors determine overall skeletal size and skeletal growth, they also play an important role in determining its specific growth and development. They are also largely responsible for the sex and ethnic differences in bone growth and mineralization. Genetic factors affecting skeletal growth and calcium metabolism probably do so by directly affecting specific metabolic or enzymatic processes. In general, genetic factors are mediated by the various hormonal factors discussed below.

The effects of various environmental factors potentially influencing skeletal growth and calcium metabolism are not completely defined. These include emotional and psychological factors, acute and chronic illnesses, socioeconomic factors, and dietary factors. This paper will not discuss any of these in detail, with the exception of dietary factors, since they impact on the calcium nutritional status of children.

HORMONAL FACTORS

Parathyroid Hormone

Though the results are somewhat contradictory, in general serum concentrations of parathyroid hormone (PTH) in children are similar to or higher than adult levels (14,15) (Fig. 1). The exact values vary with the type of PTH assay used. As in adults, the normal inverse relationship between ionized calcium and PTH has been demonstrated. Also, age-dependent changes in serum PTH concentration have been noted, with the highest values reported in the youngest children, a nadir occurring at 7–9 years of age, and a moderate rise in early adolescence (prior to the prepubertal growth spurt) (16). PTH returns to the adult normal serum value by about 20 years of age (16) (Fig. 1). There is no difference between the sexes until adolescence, when values in girls tend to be higher during the growth spurt compared with that in boys (16).

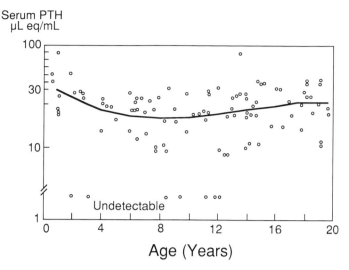

FIG. 1. Serum parathyroid (*PTH*) concentrations over time in children and adolescents. (From Arnaud et al., ref. 14, with permission.)

Vitamin D

Serum concentrations of 25-hydroxyvitamin D, thought to reflect overall vitamin D status, are essentially the same as adult values in children and adolescents (17,18) (Fig. 2). There are no differences with increasing age after the newborn period, and no sexual differences have been reported (17,19). As with adults, seasonal differences in 25-hydroxyvitamin D have been reported, with higher serum concentrations in summer than in winter (17,20).

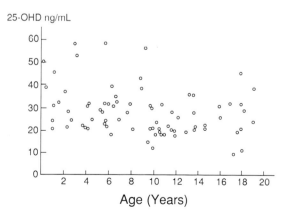

FIG. 2. Serum 25-hydroxy vitamin D (*25-OHD*) concentrations over time in children and adolescents. (From Lund et al., ref. 18, with permission.)

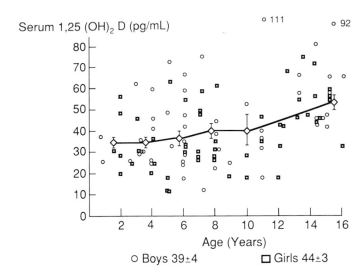

FIG. 3. Serum 1,25-dihydroxy vitamin D [*1,25(OH)₂D*] concentrations over time in children and adolescents. (From Chesney et al., ref. 21, with permission.)

Concentrations of 1,25-dihydroxyvitamin D (1,25(OH)₂D) are reported to be the same or greater than adult values in both children and adolescents (17,18,21,22) (Fig. 3). Serum concentrations of 1,25(OH)₂D have been reported to peak in adolescence in both boys and girls (23,24). In children, higher concentrations of 1,25(OH)₂D correlate positively with skeletal growth velocity (22). No study to date has reported gender differences with 1,25(OH)₂D (19), and, unlike 25O-HD, there is no seasonal variation (17,20).

Calcitonin

Though the exact physiologic role of calcitonin is unknown, it may participate in the mineralization process of bone and help to maintain skeletal integrity (25). Serum calcitonin concentrations are very high in infants and decrease with increasing age, but still remain higher than adult values throughout childhood (26,27) (Fig. 4).

Growth Hormone and Insulin-Like Growth Factors

Growth hormone is a very important modulator of human growth, and growth hormone and insulin-like growth factors (somatomedins) play an essential role in skeletal growth and calcium metabolism (28,29). For instance, it is known that growth hormone-deficient children have osteopenia, which improves after growth hormone therapy (30). Animal studies have indicated that growth hormone increases bone mass by increasing endosteal new bone formation, as well as increasing calcium

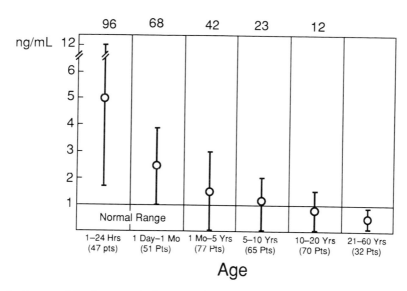

FIG. 4. Serum calcitonin concentrations over time in children and adolescents. Percent of subjects with calcitonin level above normal range. (From Samaan et al., ref. 26, with permission.)

incorporation into bone while activating intestinal absorption and inhibiting urinary calcium excretion (31,32). Thus, some of the effects of growth hormone on mineral metabolism may be manifested by its effects on the kidney. One of the first recognized effects of growth hormone in humans was a reduction in urinary phosphorous excretion (33). Studies in adult volunteers have demonstrated that growth hormone can raise serum phosphate by increasing the maximal tubular reabsorption of phosphate (34). One study has also shown hypercalcemia in children treated with growth hormone (35), although this finding was not confirmed in subsequent studies (36,37).

Although the effect of growth hormone on PTH secretion remains controversial, three studies in children treated with growth hormone have demonstrated no significant changes in serum PTH concentration (36–38). In children receiving growth hormone replacement therapy, conflicting data exist as to the effect of growth hormone on plasma 1,25(OH)$_2$D concentrations (36–39). Overall, it would appear that there is a minimal or short-lived effect. Regarding calcium absorption, increased absorption may occur in patients with acromegaly (40,41), as well as in patients treated with growth hormone (38,41).

Sex Steroids

Adolescence is characterized by marked changes in serum sex steroid concentrations as well as important increases in skeletal stature and BMC of both trabecular and cortical bone. The importance of sex steroids to normal skeletal development during adolescence is illustrated by the abnormally low bone mineral content in estrogen-deficient patients with Turner's syndrome (42), as well as decreased bone mass in hypogonadal males with testosterone deficiency (43,44). In tall boys treated with testosterone, an increase in bone density has been described (45). Excess endogenous androgen production in young women has also been associated with increased bone density (46).

Changes in mineral metabolism in adolescents are evidenced by early increases in serum alkaline phosphatase, serum phosphorous, and serum $1,25(OH)_2D$ (23). Maximal serum concentration of testosterone is achieved concurrently with the maximal rise in alkaline phosphatase, and this precedes the maximal rise in BMC by 5–10 months (10). Thus, changes in mineral metabolism occur in adolescence before the greatest changes in growth velocity and bone density, providing the necessary materials for bone growth and maturation. These changes involve the pubertal surges of testosterone in males. The exact relationship between sex steroids and PTH and/or $1,25(OH)_2D$ is unclear, but it seems likely that testosterone affects $1,25(OH)_2$ production (24). In chicks, chronic estrogen treatment allows testosterone and progesterone to increase $1,25(OH)_2D$ formation (47).

Thyroxine

Hypothyroidism is known to retard bone growth and delay the appearance of epiphyseal centers of ossification. It has been suggested that the main influence of thyroxine is to advance skeletal maturation, while that of growth hormone is to stimulate skeletal growth without advancing skeletal maturation (4). Although thyroxine plays a role in skeletal accretion of calcium, in excess (hyperthyroid subjects) it promotes reabsorption of calcium from bone and may even decrease intestinal absorption of calcium (1).

CALCIUM AVAILABILITY AND CONSERVATION

After the neonatal period, the normal values for total serum calcium are slightly higher than those of adults. Children 6 months to 2 years of age have the highest total serum calcium concentration (10.2 mg/dl), which falls to 9.8 mg/dl by 6–8 years and reaches the adult value (9.6 mg/dl) by ages 16–20 years (14) (Fig. 5). Ionized calcium values fall from 4.59 mg/dl at ages 6–12 years to an adult value of 4.22 mg/dl by 16–20 years (14). Serum calcium concentrations in children are maintained by the concerted action of a number of hormones, as discussed above, as well as by intestinal absorption of dietary calcium and retention of calcium by the kidney. Ultimately, dietary calcium availability and thus the nutritional status of growing children play an important role in pediatric calcium metabolism.

Intestinal Calcium Absorption

Most of the research on the role of the gastrointestinal tract in the control of mineral metabolism has been conducted with animals. In the rat, calcium absorption is a

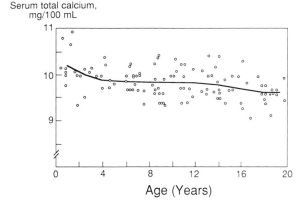

FIG. 5. Total serum calcium concentrations in children and adolescents. (From Arnaud et al., ref. 14, with permission.)

passive process until the time of weaning (3 weeks of age), after which time there is the development of active calcium absorption. Subsequent to weaning, the passive absorption of calcium declines but is still present until at least sexual maturity (6 weeks). The active process of calcium absorption peaks at about 35 days of age, when maximum growth is occurring, after which it too decreases (48). Calcium is 98 percent absorbed at 4 weeks of life, decreasing to 24 percent by 100 weeks (49) (Table 4).

Active duodenal calcium transport is a $1,25(OH)_2D$-dependent process. Significant concentrations of intestinal receptor for $1,25(OH)_2D$ do not appear until 18–28 days of life in the rat (50,51). $1,25(OH)_2D$ apparently stimulates the synthesis of intestinal calcium binding protein, the concentration of which increases dramatically at the time of weaning along with the number of $1,25(OH)_2D$ intestinal receptors (52).

Although there is little similar information about the physiology and ontogeny of calcium absorption in humans, as stated, there are some points of agreement in the

TABLE 4. *Absorption of dietary calcium by rats of various ages*

	% Ca intake	
Age (weeks)	Absorbed	Reexcreted
4	98	0.7
12	57	2
24	46	6
48–72	41	7
100	24	6

From Hansard and Crowder. (ref. 49, with permission.)

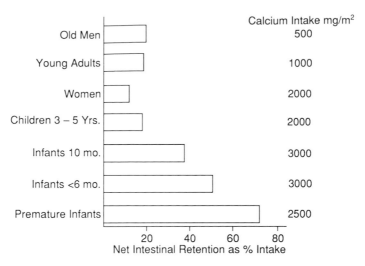

FIG. 6. Percent calcium retention and calcium intake per square meter in infants, children, and adults. (From Harrison, ref. 55, with permission.)

literature. The efficiency of absorption is increased during periods of increased calcium needs. Premature infants may absorb 75–80 percent of the ingested calcium, while as little as 15–20 percent is absorbed by adults (53–55) (Fig. 6). It is also apparent that a higher percentage of ingested calcium is absorbed at low intakes compared with high intakes. On the other hand, total amount of calcium absorbed in infants increases proportionally to the amount ingested (56,57).

Role of the Kidney in Pediatric Calcium Metabolism

Calcium homeostasis is largely regulated at the level of the intestine. Renal conservation of calcium is less important; however, if calcium appearing in the glomerular filtrate was not reabsorbed, relatively large urinary losses of calcium would occur. Ninety-eight percent of filtered calcium is reabsorbed by the renal tubules (58). However, only ionized plasma calcium and calcium complexed with various anions (60 percent of the total plasma calcium) is freely filtrable. The mitochondria of the proximal tubule of the kidney are the location of the enzyme necessary for 1 α-hydroxylation of 25-hydroxyvitamin D to make 1,25(OH)$_2$D. The activity of the 1 α-hydroxylase is controlled by hypocalcemic stimuli promoting PTH secretion. A direct effect of hypophosphatemia in stimulating 1,25(OH)$_2$D synthesis also occurs. PTH increases renal reabsorption of calcium and increases excretion of phosphate through a cyclic AMP-mediated process in the proximal renal tubule (59). Calcitonin generally stimulates calcium reabsorption by the renal tubules, although the mechanism of action is unknown. In the vitamin D-depleted state, 1,25(OH)$_2$D may increase tubular calcium reabsorption, but studies are contradictory.

An early study of calcium excretion in normal subjects found that the mean calcium excretion averaged 2 mg/kg/day at all ages in children and varied little with dietary intake (60). A later study using 24-hour urine collections to measure calcium excretion similarly reported a normal mean calcium excretion of 2.38 mg/kg/day, with an upper limit of normal of 4 mg/kg/day (61).

Dietary Intake

More than 55% of the calcium intake of the U.S. population comes from dairy products (i.e., milk, cheese, yogurt) (62). Other dietary sources of calcium include leafy green vegetables, lime-processed tortillas, and calcium-precipitated tofu. Alternative rich sources of calcium include bones, especially the soft bones of fish and tips of poultry leg bones. Dietary factors may increase calcium absorption including certain amino acids (lysine, arginine) and lactose. Other foods may decrease the absorptive efficiency of calcium, including cocoa, soy beans, kale, spinach, fiber-containing items, and bean or wheat meal, which contain hexaphosphoinositol.

The effect of inorganic phosphorus on calcium absorption remains controversial. However, excess consumption of phosphorus may contribute to the increased PTH serum concentration seen with age and the asymptomatic, but progressive osteopenia (63). Large intakes of sodium phosphate-containing carbonated beverages in adolescence may be of some concern. However, as cola soft drinks contain only about 70 mg of phosphorus/12 oz. can, two soft drinks would only contribute 12 percent of the average 1,200-mg daily phosphorus intake in adolescents (64). Perhaps a greater dietary concern regarding soft drinks is the fact that indirect evidence suggests that their intake decreases milk consumption, and thus decreases dietary calcium. Thus, there may be a greater overall effect on calcium–phosphorus metabolism.

The 1977–1978 Nationwide Food Consumption Survey reported a wide variation in calcium intake among children and adults in the United States, ranging from 530 mg for women 35–50 years old to 1,179 mg for 12–18-year-old boys (65). No group of adult females had a calcium intake equal to or greater than the RDA of 800 mg (66), again stressing the importance of calcium intake and accretion of bone mass in childhood and adolescence. A recent study in adolescent females with different calcium intakes (260 vs. 1,637 mg/d) concluded that the main determinant of calcium balance was calcium intake. As calcium intake increased, net calcium absorption increased, and urinary calcium did not change. However, this study also concluded that peak bone size, bone mass, and BMC in young women are strongly influenced by genetic information from both mothers and fathers (67). In the words of the Subcommittee on the Tenth Edition of the RDAs:

> . . . the most promising nutritional approach to reduce the risk of osteoporosis in later life is to ensure a calcium intake that allows the development of each individual's genetically programmed peak bone mass during the formative years. The importance of meeting recommended allowance at all ages is stressed, but with special attention to intakes throughout childhood to age 25 years (2).

REFERENCES

1. Royer P. Growth and development of bone tissues. In: Davis JA, Dobbing J, eds. *Scientific Foundation of Paediatrics*. London: William Heinemann Medical Books Ltd., 1974;376–399.
2. *Recommended dietary allowances*, 10th ed. Washington: National Academy Press, 1989;174–184.
3. *Calcium requirements: report of an FAO/WHO expert group*. Geneva: World Health Organization, 1962.
4. Sissons HA. The growth of bone. In: Bourne GH, ed. *The biochemistry and physiology of bone*, 2nd ed, vol III. New York: Academic Press, 1971;145–180.
5. Garn SM. The course of bone gain and the phases of bone loss. *Orthop Clin North Am* 1972;3:503–520.
6. Specker BL, Brazerol W, Tsang RC, Levin R, Searey J, Steichen J. Bone mineral content in children 1 to 6 years of age. Detectable sex differences after 4 years of age. *Am J Dis Child* 1987;141:343–344.
7. Mazess RB, Cameron JR. Skeletal growth in school children: maturation and bone mass. *Am J Phys Anthropol* 1971;35:399–408.
8. Mazess RB, Cameron JR. Growth of bone in school children: comparison of radiographic morphometry and photon absorptiometry. *Growth* 1972;36:77–92.
9. Krabbe S, Transbol I, Christiansen C. Bone mineral homeostasis, bone growth, and mineralization during years of pubertal growth: a unifying concept. *Arch Dis Child* 1982;57:359–363.
10. Krabbe S, Christiansen C, Rodbro P, Transbol I. Effect of puberty on rates of bone growth and mineralization. *Arch Dis Child* 1979;54:950–953.
11. Alvioli LV. Calcium and osteoporosis. *Annu Rev Nutr* 1984;4:471–491.
12. Roche AF. Skeletal status in normal children. In: *Osteoporosis: current concepts*. Report of the Seventh Ross Conference on Medical Research. Columbus, OH: Ross Laboratories, 1987;8–11.
13. Wakefield T Jr, Disney GW, Mason RL, Beauchene RE. Relationships among anthropometric indices of growth and creatinine and hydroxyproline excretion in preadolescent black and white girls. *Growth* 1980;44:192–204.
14. Arnaud SB, Goldsmith RS, Stickler GB, McCall JT, Arnaud CD. Serum parathyroid hormone and blood minerals: interrelationship in normal children. *Pediatr Res* 1973;7:485–493.
15. Root A, Gruskin A, Reber RM, Stopa A, Duckett G. Serum concentrations of parathyroid hormone in infants, children and adolescents. *J Pediatr* 1974;85:329–336.
16. Krabbe S, Transbol I, Christiansen C. Bone mineral homeostasis, bone growth, and mineralization during years of pubertal growth: a unifying concept. *Arch Dis Child* 1982;57:359–363.
17. Chesney RW, Rosen JF, Hamstra AJ, Smith C, Mahaffey K, DeLuca HF. Absence of seasonal variation in serum concentrations of 1,25-dihydroxyvitamin D despite a rise in 25-dihydroxyvitamin in summer. *J Clin Endocrinol Metab* 1981;53:139–142.
18. Lund B, Clausen N, Lund B, Andersen E, Sorensen OH. Age dependent variations in serum 1,25-dihydroxyvitamin D in childhood. *Acta Endocrinol* 1980;94:426–429.
19. Fujisawa Y, Kida K, Matsuda H. Role of change in vitamin D metabolism with age in calcium and phosphorus metabolism in normal human subjects. *J Clin Endocrinol Metab* 1984;59:719–726.
20. Seino Y, Shimotsiyi T, Yamaoka K, et al. Plasma 1,25-dihydroxyvitamin D concentration in cords, newborns, infants and children. *Calcif Tissue Int* 1980;30:1–3.
21. Chesney RW, Rosen JF, Hamstra AJ, DeLuca HF. Serum 1,25-dihydroxy vitamin D levels in normal children and in vitamin D disorders. *Am J Dis Child* 1980;134:135–139.
22. Taylor AF, Norman ME. Vitamin D metabolite levels in normal children. *Pediatr Res* 1984;18:886–890.
23. Aksnes L, Aarskog D. Plasma concentrations of vitamin D metabolites in puberty: effect of sexual maturation and implication for growth. *J Clin Endocrinol Metab* 1982;55:94–101.
24. Krabbe S, Hummer L, Christiansen C. Serum levels of vitamin D metabolites and testosterone in male puberty. *J Clin Endocrinol Metab* 1986;62:503–507.
25. Austin LA, Heath H. Calcitonin. *N Engl J Med* 1981;304:269–278.
26. Samaan N, Anderson GD, Adam-Mazne ME. Immunoreactive calcitonin in the mother, neonate, child, and adult. *Am J Obstet Gynecol* 1975;121:622–625.
27. Klein GL, Wadlington EL, Collins ED, Catherwood BD, Deftos LJ. Calcitonin levels in sera of infants and children: relations to age and periods of bone growth. *Calcif Tissue Int* 1984;36:635–638.
28. Rechler MM, Nissley SP, Roth J. Hormonal regulation of human growth. *N Engl J Med* 1987;316:941–943.

29. Thorner MO, Vance ML. Growth hormone, 1988. *J Clin Invest* 1988;82:745–747.
30. Shore RM, Chesney RW, Mazess RB, Rose PG, Bargman GJ. Bone mineral status in growth hormone deficiency. *J Pediatr* 1980;96:393–396.
31. Harris WH, Heaney RP, Jowsey J, et al. Growth hormone: the effect on skeletal renewal in the adult dog. 1. Morphometric studies. *Calcif Tissue Res* 1972;10:1–3.
32. Heaney RP, Harris WH, Cockin J, Weinberg EH. Growth hormone: the effect on skeletal renewal in the adult dog II. Mineral kinetic studies. *Calcif Tissue Res* 1972;10:14–22.
33. Hennemen PH, Forbes AP, Moldawer M, Dempsey EF, Carrol EL. Effects of growth hormone in man. *J Clin Invest* 1960;39:1223–1238.
34. Corvilain J, Abramow M. Some effects of human growth hormone on renal hemodynamics and on tubular phosphate transport in man. *J Clin Invest* 1962;41:1230–1235.
35. Bryson MF, Forbes GB, Amirhakimi GH, Reina JC. Metabolic response to growth hormone administration, with particular reference to the occurrence of hypercalciuria. *Pediatr Res* 1972;6:743–751.
36. Gertner JM, Horst RL, Broadus AE, Rasmussen H, Genel M. Parathyroid function and vitamin D metabolism during human growth hormone replacement. *J Clin Endocrinol Metab* 1979;49:185–188.
37. Gertner JM, Tamborlane WV, Hintz RL, Horst RL, Genel M. The effects on mineral metabolism of overnight growth hormone infusion in growth hormone deficiency. *J Clin Endocrinol Metab* 1981;53:818–822.
38. Chipman JJ, Zerwekh J, Nicar M, Marks J, Pak CYC. Effect of growth hormone administration: reciprocal changes in serum 1 alpha-25-dihydroxyvitamin D and intestinal calcium absorption. *J Clin Endocrinol Metab* 1980;51:321–324.
39. Burstein S, Chen IW, Tsang RC. Effects of growth hormone replacement therapy on 1,25-dihydroxyvitamin D and calcium metabolism. *J Clin Endocrinol Metab* 1983;56:1246–1251.
40. Takamoto S, Tsuchiya H, Onishi T, et al. Changes in calcium homeostasis in acromegaly treated by pituitary adenomectomy. *J Clin Endocrinol Metab* 1985;61:7–11.
41. Hanna S, Harrison MT, MacIntyre I, Fraser R. Effects of growth hormone on calcium and magnesium metabolism. *Br Med J* 1961;3:12–15.
42. Brown DM, Jowsey J, Phil, D, Bradford DS. Osteoporosis in ovarian dysgenesis. *J Pediatr* 1974;84:816–820.
43. Finkelstein JS, Klibanski A, Neer RM, Greenspan SL, Rosenthal DI, Crowley WF Jr. Osteoporosis in men with idiopathic hypogonadotropic hypogonadism. *Ann Intern Med* 1987;106:354–361.
44. Smith DAS, Walker MS. Changes in plasma steroids and bone density in Kleinfelter's syndrome. *Calcif Tissue Res* 1976;22:225–228.
45. Exner GU, Prader A, Elsasser U, Anliker M. Effects of high dose estrogen and testosterone treatment in adolescents upon trabecular and compact bone mass measured by I^{125} computed tomography. A preliminary study. *Acta Endocrinol* 1980;94:126–131.
46. Buchanan JR, Hospodar P, Myers C, Leuenberger P, Demers LM. Effect of excess endogenous androgens on bone density in young women. *J Clin Endocrinol Metab* 1988;67:937–943.
47. Pike JW, Spanos E, Colston KW, MacIntyre I, Haussler MR. Influence of estrogen on renal vitamin D hydroxylases and serum $1,25(OH)_2D_3$ in chicks. *Am J Physiol* 1978;235:E338–E343.
48. Dostal LA, Toverud SU. Effect of vitamin D_3 on duodenal calcium absorption in vivo during early development. *Am J Physiol* 1984;246:G528–G534.
49. Hansard SL, Crowder HM. The physiological behavior of calcium in the rat. *J Nutr* 1957;62:325–339.
50. Halloran BP, DeLuca HF. Appearance of the intestinal cytosolic receptor for 1,25-dihydroxyvitamin D_3 during neonatal development in the rat. *J Biol Chem* 1981;256:7338–7342.
51. Pierce EA, DeLuca HF. Regulation of the intestinal 1,25-dihydroxyvitamin D_3 receptor during neonatal development in the rat. *Arch Biochem Biophys* 1988;261:241–249.
52. Bruns MEH, Bruns DE, Alvioli LV. Vitamin D-dependent calcium-binding protein of rat intestine: changes during postnatal development sensitivity to 1,25-dihydroxycholecalciferol. *Endocrinology* 1979;105:934–938.
53. Heaney RP, Sarille PD, Recker RR. Calcium absorption as a function of calcium intake. *J Lab Clin Med* 1975;85:881–890.
54. Heaney RP, Gallagher JC, Johnston CC, Neer R, Parfitt AM, Whedon GD. Calcium nutrition and bone health in the elderly. *Am J Clin Nutr* 1982;36:986–1013.
55. Harrison HE. Factors influencing calcium absorption. *Fed Proc* 1959;18:1085–1092.
56. Kahn B, Straub CP, Robbins PJ. Retention of radiostrontium, strontium, calcium and phosphorus by infants. *Pediatrics* 1969;43:651–667.

57. Younoszai MK. Development of intestinal calcium transport. In: Lebenthal E, ed. *Textbook of gastroenterology and nutrition in infancy*. New York: Raven Press, 1981;623–629.
58. Chesney RW, Zelikovic I. The metabolism of vitamin D and the renal handling of calcium and phosphate. In: Castells S, Finberg L, eds. *Metabolic bone disease in children*. New York: Marcel Dekker, 1990;43–70.
59. Johnson V, Spitzer A. Renal reabsorption of phosphate during development: whole-kidney events. *Am J Physiol* 1986;251:F251–F256.
60. Knapp EL. Factors influencing the urinary excretion of calcium. 1. In normal persons. *J Clin Invest* 1947;26:182–202.
61. Ghazali S, Barratt TM. Urinary excretion of calcium and magnesium in children. *Arch Dis Child* 1974;49:97–101.
62. Block G, Dresser CM, Hartman AM, Carroll MD. Nutrient sources in the American diet: quantitative data from the NHANES II survey. I. Vitamins and minerals. *Am J Epidemiol* 1985;122:13–26.
63. Reiss E, Canterbury JM, Bercovitz MA, Kaplan EL. The role of phosphate in the secretion of parathyroid hormone in man. *J Clin Invest* 1970;49:2146–2149.
64. Massey LK, Strang MM. Soft drink consumption, phosphorus intake, and osteoporosis. *J Am Diet Assoc* 1982;80:581–583.
65. USDA. *Nationwide Food Consumption Survey. Nutrient intakes: individuals in 48 states, year 1977–78*. Report no. 1-2, Consumer Nutrition Division, Human Nutrition Information Service. Hyattsville, MD: U.S. Department of Agriculture. 1984.
66. USDA. *Nationwide Food Consumption Survey. Continuing survey of food intakes of individuals. Women 19–50 years and their children 1–5 years, 4 days, 1985*. Report no. 85-4. Hyattsville, MD: Nutrition Monitoring Division, Human Nutrition Information Service, 1987.
67. Matkovic V, Fontana D, Tominac C, Goel P, Chesnut CH III. Factors that influence peak bone mass formation: a study of calcium balance and the inheritance of bone mass in adolescent females. *Am J Clin Nutr* 1990;52:878–888.

Calcium Nutriture for Mothers and Children, edited by
Reginald C. Tsang and Francis Mimouni. Carnation
Nutrition Education Series, Vol. 3. Carnation Co.,
Glendale/Raven Press, Ltd., New York © 1992.

Calcium Metabolism in the Pregnant and Lactating Female

Roy M. Pitkin

*Department of Obstetrics and Gynecology, UCLA School of Medicine,
Los Angeles, California 90024-1740*

Pregnancy and lactation represent two stages of the reproductive cycle that have profound implications with respect to calcium homeostasis. Each is characterized by substantial loss of calcium, across the placenta in the one case and via the breast in the other. These losses must be balanced by increased absorption and/or diminished excretion if the skeleton is to be maintained in optimal status. The purpose of this chapter is to review the literature with respect to calcium metabolism in the pregnant and lactating woman and to summarize the current understanding of calcium homeostasis during these two states.

PREGNANCY

The sites of calcium accumulation during pregnancy are listed in Table 1. The total incremental accumulation at term averages about 30 g, almost all of it in the fetal skeleton. Placental calcification represents a small and quite variable amount. Minimal levels are found in fetal tissues other than bone and in expanded maternal fluids and tissues.

Maternal Adjustments

Faced with the need to provide for fetal growth and development and at the same time preserve her own homeostasis, the pregnant woman undergoes a remarkable series of physiologic adjustments (1). Many of these adjustments have implications with respect to calcium metabolism. Gastrointestinal motility slows, renal function increases, and extracellular fluid volume expands. Although mineralization of the fetal skeleton occurs predominantly during the last third of intrauterine life, maternal adaptation seems to begin much earlier. Intestinal absorption of calcium increases during early gestation, and calcium balance is generally positive (2). Gertner and associates (3) found that calcium tolerance tests caused increased calciuric and cal-

27

TABLE 1. *Calcium accumulation in pregnancy at term*

Site	Average (g)
Fetus	28.4
Placenta	1.0
Amniotic fluid	0.2
Maternal extracellular fluid Maternal uterus and breasts	Minimal
Total	~30

cemic responses in pregnant women compared with the same subjects postpartum, leading to the characterization of pregnancy as a "state of physiologic hypercalciuria." Others (4), however, have concluded from the close correlation between calcium excretion and creatinine clearance that the gestational increase in glomerular filtration rate is responsible.

That the maternal serum total calcium concentration declines with pregnancy has been recognized for many years. The fall is more or less progressive to a nadir in the mid-third trimester, with a slight rise thereafter (Fig. 1) (5). The pattern parallels that of serum albumin (Fig. 2), the principal binding protein of calcium, and ionic calcium concentrations remain constant (6). Serum calcium changes with gestation appear independent of dietary intake.

The effect of pregnancy on endocrine regulation of calcium metabolism has been the subject of considerable study. Theoretically, increased parathyroid hormone se-

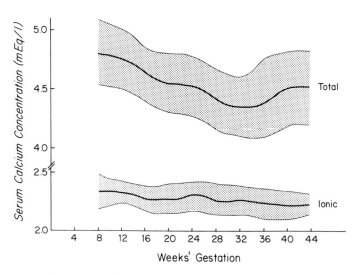

FIG. 1. Mean (±2 SD) total and ionic calcium concentrations. (From Pitkin and Gebhardt, ref. 6, with permission.)

cretion would represent a logical maternal adjustment to the expanding maternal extracellular fluid volume, increased urinary excretion, and placental calcium transfer. A number of studies over the past 20 years have found increased parathyroid hormone levels at some stage of gestation (Fig. 3), leading to the traditional view of pregnancy as a state of ''physiologic hyperparathyroidism'' (7). However, this characterization has been challenged recently by several recent investigations (8–12), generally using more specific assay systems, which have found no gestational increase, and in some cases an actual decrease (Table 2) in blood levels of parathyroid hormone. Less studied, though equally unsettled, is the influence of pregnancy on calcitonin secretion (7–9).

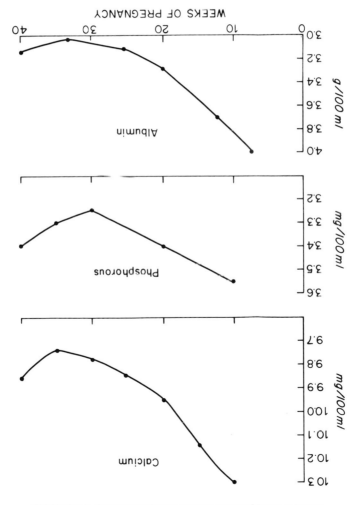

FIG. 2. Mean total calcium, phosphorous, and albumin concentrations in pregnancy. (From Pitkin, ref. 5, with permission.)

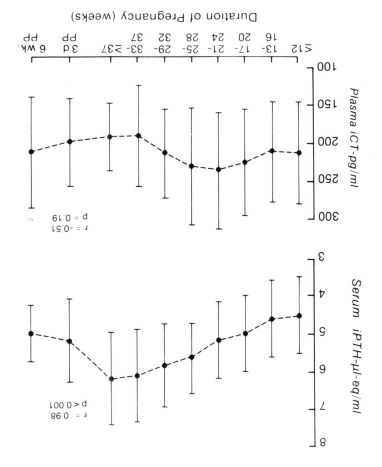

FIG. 3. Mean (± 2 SD) immunoreactive parathyroid hormone (*iPTH*) and calcitonin (*iCT*) concentrations in pregnancy and postpartum (*pp*). (From Pitkin et al., ref. 7, with permission.)

TABLE 2. *Parathyroid hormone in pregnancy*[a]

	Mean $\pm$ SD (ng/L)
Nonpregnant	24.8 $\pm$ 9.0
First trimester	12.9 $\pm$ 5.0
Second trimester	16.0 $\pm$ 6.0
Third trimester	13.5 $\pm$ 7.0

[a] Measured by immunoradiometric assay for intact hormone; data at Davis et al., ref. 10.

The situation is somewhat clearer with respect to vitamin D. The principal circulating form, 25-hydroxyvitamin D_3 (25-OHD$_3$), is generally unaffected by pregnancy, and levels reflect exposure to ultraviolet light, as well as dietary intake. However, the biologically active form, 1,25-dihydroxyvitamin D_3 [1,25(OH)$_2$D$_3$], increases during pregnancy and by term the serum concentration is approximately doubled (12–16). Although placenta and/or decidua as well as the fetal kidney produce 1,25(OH)$_2$D$_3$, the source of the increased maternal blood levels is more likely increased 1α-hydroxylation in the maternal kidney (17). Whatever the source, it seems clear that an increase in circulating 1,25(OH)$_2$D$_3$ levels plays a key role in the maternal adaptive process. It almost surely is responsible for an improvement in intestinal absorption of calcium and it probably is involved in maintaining ionic calcium within its characteristically narrow physiologic range in extracellular fluid.

Maternal Skeleton

Calcium stored in the adult female skeleton averages a little more than 1 kg and is available at times of increased need such as pregnancy. Even if there were no calcium intake, the "cost" of a pregnancy would represent only less than 3 percent of the skeletal stores.

What happens to maternal bone density during pregnancy has been the subject of several investigations. Lemke and colleagues (18), using x-ray spectrophometry during the second trimester and again postpartum, described a pregnancy-associated loss in trabecular but not in cortical bone. Christiansen et al. (19) found no change in radial bone mineral content in women studied at four points during gestation. Sowers and associates (20), using dual photon absorptiometry, found no significant change in femoral bone mineral content between preconceptional and puerperal studies. Thus, there seems to be a reasonable consensus that there is little effect of gestation, at least on long bones. However, the failure to control for calcium intake is an important limitation of all reports appearing thus far.

A fascinating study, if for no other reason than its uniqueness, is that of Purdie and associates (21), who analyzed bone biopsy specimens histologically and biochemically from three groups of subjects, at 8–10 weeks' gestation, at 39–40 weeks' gestation, and nonpregnant controls. Early gestation was characterized by evidence of increased bone resorption, whereas near term there was active bone formation and rapid mineralization with minimal resorption. These findings are generally opposite to what has been postulated from noninvasive studies.

Dietary Allowance and Supplementation

The Recommended Dietary Allowance (RDA) for calcium is 1,200 mg/day for women aged 11–24 years and 800 mg/day for older women (22). During pregnancy the RDA is 1,200 mg/day irrespective of age. Apparently normal pregnancy occurs in many circumstances at calcium intakes substantially below the RDA, a situation that may reflect either an adaptive improvement in intestinal absorption or subsidization by bone demineralization. For whatever reason, there seem to be few adverse effects of low calcium intake. However, young women in whom bone mineralization may not be complete could represent a particularly vulnerable group, and the Food and Nutrition Board's Committee on Nutritional Status during Pregnancy and Lactation (23) recommends that gravidas under age 25 who have a low calcium intake be considered for supplementation (at a level of 600 mg/day). For older gravidas who do not ordinarily consume an adequate diet, supplementation of 250 mg/day is advised.

Vitamin D is unique among essential nutrients because, while it comes from dietary sources, it can also be synthesized in the skin. The latter source is clearly the major one. The RDA for vitamin D is 10 μg (400 IU) up to age 25 and 5 μg (200 IU) afterwards (22). It is also 10 μg (400 IU) during pregnancy. A supplement of 10 μg per day is advised for complete vegetarians and one of 5 μg per day for other women whose intake of vitamin D-fortified milk is low, especially those in northern latitudes during winter (23).

The practice of routine supplementation of vitamins and minerals during pregnancy is widespread. In the case of vitamin D, routine supplementation is very common in Europe, where vitamin D deficiency occurs occasionally. Studies have suggested beneficial efforts of routine vitamin D supplementation on birth weight, neonatal calcium homeostasis, and maternal bone health (24,25).

Fetal and Placental Relationships

The central feature of fetal calcium physiology is the placenta's ability to transmit calcium ions actively from mother to fetus against a concentration gradient, making the fetus (at least during the last third of intrauterine life) relatively hypercalcemic. This situation would be expected to result in suppression of parathyroid hormone secretion and/or stimulation of calcitonin release. The evidence regarding these endocrinologic relationships is conflicting, but most studies have not found parathyroid hormone concentrations in cord blood to be suppressed (1). Calcitonin concentration does seem to be increased in fetal blood, suggesting that this hormone may play a role in fetal growth and development.

The principal circulating form of vitamin D, 25-OHD$_3$, apparently crosses the placenta readily. Maternal and fetal levels correlate positively with fetal values 20–30% below maternal. However, maternal and fetal levels of 1,25(OH)$_2$D$_3$ do not correlate. This lack of correlation suggests a lack of placental transfer of 1,25(OH)$_2$D$_3$, although direct studies in sheep suggest otherwise (26). The relationship is complicated by the ability of both the placenta and the fetal kidney to produce the hormone. Theoretically, there would seem to be relatively little need for 1,25(OH)$_2$D$_3$ in the fetus because its calcium supply is regulated by the placenta. Figure 4 summarizes the relationships between mother, fetus, and newborn.

The effect of maternal calcium–vitamin D nutriture on fetal growth and devel-

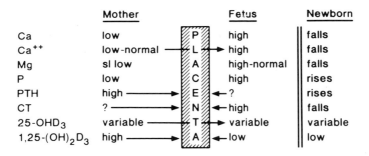

	Mother		Fetus	Newborn
Ca	low	P	high	falls
Ca++	low-normal →	L →	high	falls
Mg	sl low	A	high-normal	falls
P	low	C	high	rises
PTH	high ——→	E ←	?	rises
CT	? ——→	N ←	high	falls
25-OHD₃	variable ——→	T →	variable	variable
1,25-(OH)₂D₃	high ——→	A ←	low	low

FIG. 4. Schematic model of calcium homeostasis in the pregnant woman, fetus, and newborn infant. *PTH,* parathyroid hormone; *CT,* calcitonin. (From Pitkin, ref. 1, with permission.)

opment is not known with certainty. In general, no consistent effect of maternal dietary deficiency has been found, suggesting some degree of fetal protection by maternal stores and/or the placental transport mechanism. Individual reports have suggested that maternal vitamin D deficiency may lead to neonatal hypocalcemia and enamel hypoplasia (24,27).

Clinical Aspects

The gestational needs for calcium are high enough that milk or milk products are required to meet them if diet is to be the only source. Individuals with lactose intolerance may not be able to consume these high intakes without serious effects. Fortunately, there is a tendency for lactose intolerance to improve during gestation (28), so a previously intolerant gravida may be able to sustain an adequate milk intake. Dairy foods high in calcium but low in lactose, such as cheese and yogurt, may be helpful. If necessary, supplemental calcium should be given.

A common problem in late pregnancy is episodic, usually nocturnal, cramping of the calf muscles. Traditionally this has been thought to reflect transient hypocalcemia, presumably related to excessive phosphate intake. The standard treatments include reduction of milk intake and substitution of a nonphosphate salt of calcium or ingestion of aluminum-containing antacids (to inhibit phosphate absorption by precipitating insoluble aluminum phosphate compounds). Although these theories seem logical, attempts to confirm them experimentally have proved disappointing, and definition of the relationships among leg cramps, calcium, milk, and antacids remains elusive (29,30).

Much interest over the past decade has centered on a possible relationship between calcium intake and acute hypertensive disorders of pregnancy. The first evidence came from epidemiologic considerations (31), and subsequent randomized trials have indicated that calcium supplementation lowers blood pressure in normal gravidas acutely (32). Clinical studies are currently under way to test the ability of calcium supplementation to prevent preeclampsia. The relationships between calcium status and hypertension in the pregnant woman are detailed in the chapter by Myatt.

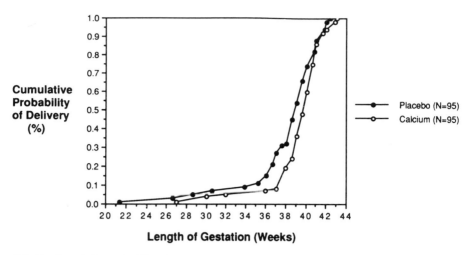

FIG. 5. Cumulative probability of delivery in calcium-supplemented and control subjects (life table analysis). (From Repke et al., ref 32, with permission.)

A beneficial effect of calcium supplementation on preterm birth has also been suggested (33). In a double-blind randomized trial involving adolescent gravidas, those given calcium supplements (2 g of elemental calcium as calcium carbonate) had significantly lower frequencies of preterm delivery (7.4 percent vs. 21.1 percent), spontaneous labor and preterm delivery (6.4 percent vs. 17.9 percent), and low birth weight (9.6 percent vs. 21.1 percent). Furthermore, calcium produced a shift in the probability of delivery toward longer gestation (Fig. 5).

LACTATION

Breastfeeding also poses distinct implications for maternal calcium metabolism. The amount of calcium secreted in milk actually exceeds that transferred by the placenta, implying a greater dietary need for and/or enhanced efficiency of absorption and/or more subsidization from maternal stores. On the other hand, lactation does not seem to be associated with certain types of adjustments affecting calcium balance, such as expansion of extracellular volume and increased glomerular filtration.

Transfer to Milk

Calcium is transferred directly from serum to milk (33). The mean (±SD) concentration in mature milk is 280 (±26) mg/l. About two-thirds of the calcium in human milk is bound to casein, and the remainder exists as a soluble citrate complex. The concentration of calcium in milk seems to be closely regulated, and there is little evidence of a relationship with maternal nutritional status.

Vitamin D is also transferred directly from serum to milk (34). Its level averages 0.55 (± 0.1) µg/l in the human. In contrast to calcium, milk vitamin D activity correlates directly with maternal vitamin D status. Milk concentrations can fall to undetectable levels in cases of maternal deficiency, leading to rickets in the infant who depends solely on dietary sources. Furthermore, high and potentially toxic amounts can appear in milk with maternal overdosage.

Assuming daily milk production of 600 ml, as would be usual at about 3 months postpartum, about 168 mg of calcium and 0.33 µg of vitamin D would be excreted in milk each day. With a daily production of 1 l, as would be customary at 6 months, the values become 280 mg and 0.55 µg, respectively.

Maternal Physiology

It is generally assumed that calcium absorption improves during lactation as part of the adaptation to increased need. If this is the case, it is probably mediated through 1,25(OH)$_2$D$_3$ augmentation, as some studies have found serum levels of this hormone to be increased in the lactating woman (34). Specker and associates (35) studied lactation in relation to vegetarian and omnivorous diet; 1,25(OH)$_2$D$_3$ levels were higher in lactators than in nonlactators and in omnivores than in vegetarians.

The effect of lactation on bone density has received a great deal of attention because of the obvious implications regarding bone health in both the short and long term. Unfortunately, most of these studies have been cross-sectional rather than longitudinal, have paid little if any attention to calcium intake, and have relied entirely on history for data about breastfeeding. With these caveats, research generally indicates some acute loss of bone mineral during lactation (34); it is unclear to what extent this finding reflects simply the obvious excretion into milk or whether the hypoestrogenism accompanying lactation is also involved. There appears to be prompt remineralization with weaning, which probably accounts for a failure in remote studies to find a correlation between prior lactation and bone density. Furthermore, bone mineral estimations and tabulations of fracture occurrence in older women have not usually been found to relate to a history of breastfeeding.

Dietary Allowances and Supplementation

The RDA for calcium during lactation is 1,200 mg, irrespective of age, which represents an increase of 400 mg for the 25 year and over age group (22). The RDA for vitamin D during lactation is 10 µg for all ages, a doubling of the allowance for women over 25.

The increased calcium and vitamin D needs with lactation can be met by the appropriate diet, and the Committee on Nutritional Status during Pregnancy and Lactation recommends this as the appropriate means (34). For women whose eating patterns lead to a low intake of one or more nutrients and for whom dietary adjustments are not feasible, nutritional supplements may be appropriate.

REFERENCES

1. Pitkin RM. Calcium metabolism in pregnancy and the perinatal period: a review. *Am J Obstet Gynecol* 1985;151:99–109.
2. Heaney RP, Skillman TG. Calcium metabolism in normal pregnancy. *J Clin Endocrinol Metab* 1971;33:661–670.
3. Gertner JM, Coustan DR, Kliger AS, Mallette LE, Ravin N, Broadus AE. Pregnancy as state of physiologic absorptive hypercalciuria. *Am J Med* 1986;81:451–456.
4. Howarth AT, Morgan DB, Payne RB. Urinary excretion of calcium in late pregnancy and its relation to creatinine clearance. *Am J Obstet Gynecol* 1977;129:499–502.
5. Pitkin RM. Calcium metabolism in pregnancy: a review. *Am J Obstet Gynecol* 1975;121:724–737.
6. Pitkin RM, Gebhardt MP. Serum calcium concentrations in human pregnancy. *Am J Obstet Gynecol* 1977;127:775–778.
7. Pitkin RM, Reynolds WA, Williams GA, Hargis GK. Calcium metabolism in pregnancy: a longitudinal study. *Am J Obstet Gynecol* 1979;133:781–787.
8. Whitehead M, Lane G, Young O, et al. Interrelationships of calcium-regulating hormones during normal pregnancy. *Br Med J* 1981;3:10–12.
9. Pedersen EB, Johannesen P, Kristensen S, et al. Calcium, parathyroid hormone and calcitonin in normal pregnancy and preeclampsia. *Gynecol Obstet Invest* 1984;18:156–164.
10. Davis OK, Hawkins DS, Rubin LP, Posillico JT, Brown EM, Schiff I. Serum parathyroid hormone (PTH) in pregnant women determined by an immunoradiometric assay for intact PTH. *J Clin Endocrinol Metab* 1988;67:850–852.
11. Salinas M, Martinez ME, Catalan P, Ordas J, Navarro P. Biochemical parameters of calcium metabolism in pregnant women: influence of milk supplementation. *Nutrition* 1987;3:407–411.
12. Mimouni F, Tsang RC, Hertzberg VS, Neumann V, Ellis K. Parathyroid hormone and calcitriol changes in normal and insulin-dependent diabetic pregnancies. *Obstet Gynecol* 1989;74:49–54.
13. Kumar R, Cohen WR, Silva P, Epstein FH. Elevated 1,25-dihydroxyvitamin D plasma levels in normal human pregnancy and lactation. *J Clin Invest* 1979;63:342–344.
14. Bouillon R, Van Assche FA, Van Baelen H, Heyns W, De Moor P. Influence of the vitamin D-binding protein on the serum concentration of 1,25-dihydroxyvitamin D_3. *J Clin Invest* 1981;67:589–596.
15. Reddy GS, Norman AW, Willis DM, et al. Regulation of vitamin D metabolism in normal human pregnancy. *J Clin Endocrinol Metab* 1983;56:363–370.
16. Markestad T, Ulstein M, Aksnes L, Aarskog D. Serum concentrations of vitamin D metabolites in vitamin D supplemental pregnant women. A longitudinal study. *Acta Obstet Gynecol Scand* 1986;65:63–67.
17. Turner M, Barre PE, Benjamin A, Goltzman D, Gascon-Barre M. Does the maternal kidney contribute to the increased circulating 1,25-dihydroxyvitamin D concentrations during pregnancy? *Mineral Electrolyte Metab* 1988;14:246–252.
18. Lamke B, Brundin J, Moberg P. Changes of bone mineral content during pregnancy and lactation. *Acta Obstet Gynecol Scand* 1977;56:217–219.
19. Christianson C, Rodbro P, Heinild B. Unchanged total body calcium in normal human pregnancy. *Acta Obstet Gynecol Scand* 1976;55:141–143.
20. Sowers MF, Crutchfield M, Jannausch M, Updike S, Corton G. A prospective evaluation of bone mineral change in pregnancy. *Obstet Gynecol* 1991;77:841–845.
21. Purdie DW, Aaron JE, Selby PL. Bone histology and mineral homeostasis in human pregnancy. *Br J Obstet Gynaecol* 1988;95:849–854.
22. National Research Council. Recommended Dietary Allowance, (10th ed.) Washington, DC: National Academy Press, 1989.
23. Institute of Medicine. Committee on Nutritional Status during Pregnancy and Lactation. *Nutrition during pregnancy: I. Weight gain. II. Nutrient supplements.* Washington, DC: National Academy Press, 1990.
24. Brooke OG, Brown IRF, Bone CDM, et al. Vitamin D supplements in pregnant Asian women: effects on calcium status and fetal growth. *Br Med J* 1980;280:751–754.
25. Marya RK, Rathee S, Dua V, Sangwan K. Effect of vitamin D supplementation during pregnancy on foetal growth. *Indian J Med Res* 1988;88:488–492.
26. Devaskar UP, Ho M, Devaskar SU, Tsang RC. 25-hydroxy- and Iα-dihydroxyvitamin D. Maternal-

fetal relationship and the transfer of 1,25-dyhydroxyvitamin D_3 across the placenta in an ovine model. *Dev Pharmacol Ther* 1984;7:213–220.

27. Cockburn F, Belton NR, Purvis RJ, et al. Maternal vitamin D intake and mineral metabolism in mothers and their newborn infants. *Br Med J* 1980;281:11–14.

28. Villar J, Kestler E, Castillo P, Juarez A, Menendez R, Solomons N. Improved lactose digestion during pregnancy: a case of physiologic adaptation? *Obstet Gynecol* 1988;71:697–700.

29. Hammar M, Larsson L, Tegler L. Calcium treatment of leg cramps in pregnancy. *Acta Obstet Gynecol Scand* 1981;60:345–347.

30. Hammar MG, Berg G, Solheim F, Larsson L. Calcium and magnesium status in pregnant women. A comparison between treatment with calcium and vitamin C in pregnant women with leg cramps. *Int J Vitam Nutr Res* 1987;57:179–183.

31. Belizan JM, Villar J, Repke J. The relationship between calcium intake and pregnancy-induced hypertension: up-to-date evidence. *Am J Obstet Gynecol* 1988;158:898–902.

32. Repke JT, Villar J, Anderson C, Pareja G, Dubin N, Belizan JM. Biochemical changes associated with blood pressure reduction induced by calcium supplementation during pregnancy. *Am J Obstet Gynecol* 1989;160:684–690.

33. Villar J, Repke JT. Calcium supplementation during pregnancy may reduce preterm delivery in high-risk populations. *Am J Obstet Gynecol* 1990;163:1124–1131.

34. Institute of Medicine. Committee on Nutritional Status during Pregnancy and Lactation. *Nutrition during Lactation*. Washington, DC: National Academy Press, 1991.

35. Specker BL, Tsang RC, Ho M, Miller D. Effect of vegetarian diet on serum 1,25-dihydroxyvitamin D concentrations during lactation. *Obstet Gynecol* 1987;70:870–874.

Calcium Nutriture for Mothers and Children, edited by
Reginald C. Tsang and Francis Mimouni. Carnation
Nutrition Education Series, Vol. 3. Carnation Co.,
Glendale/Raven Press, Ltd., New York © 1992.

Vitamin D Functions and Requirements in the First Year of Life

Francis Mimouni

Departments of Pediatrics, Obstetrics, and Gynecology, Magee-Womens Hospital and the University of Pittsburgh School of Medicine, Pittsburgh, Pennsylvania 15213-3180

Vitamin D requirements in the first year of life are determined by rates of endogenous vitamin D production, dietary vitamin D, and vitamin D metabolism and function. In spite of significant progress in our understanding of these factors, vitamin D-deficiency rickets has not been eradicated. It is still found in developed countries such as the United States, and in some developing countries it is a major contributor to infant morbidity. In this chapter, I will review those aspects of vitamin D production and metabolism that are particularly relevant to the understanding of vitamin D deficiency. I will then review the various physiologic functions of vitamin D and the clinical and radiological consequences of its deficiency. Various mechanisms leading to deficiency will be described using typical examples from populations at risk throughout the world. I will then review the basis for current Recommended Dietary Allowances (RDAs), and the different clinical trials supporting (or not supporting) the current RDAs. I will finally conclude with a personal opinion based upon the available evidence.

VITAMIN D SYNTHESIS AND FUNCTION

Vitamin D Production in Skin

The photoproduction of vitamin D depends on the quantum of ultraviolet B (UVB) photons that penetrate the skin. Therefore, the following points are to be emphasized: the first is the *solar zenith angle*, which influences the number of UVB photons reaching the skin. The further from the equator and the closer to the earth's poles, the more UVB photons will be scattered and/or absorbed by the earth's atmosphere. Thus, geographic *latitude* and *season* are important variables that may affect vitamin D skin production in that they will affect the angle at which the sun's rays enter the atmosphere (1–3).

In a challenging study, Webb et al. (2) recently demonstrated that exposure to winter sunlight in Boston and Edmonton will not promote vitamin D_3 synthesis in

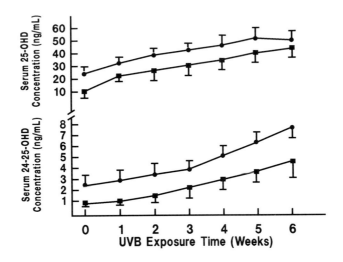

FIG. 1. Serum 25-hydroxyvitamin D (25-OHD) (*top*) and 24,25-dihydroxyvitamin D [24,25(OH)$_2$D] (*bottom*) concentrations during serial ultraviolet B (*UVB*) exposure in white (●) and black (■) subjects. Although serum 25-OHD and 24,25(OH)$_2$D concentrations were lower in blacks versus whites at entry, the subsequent increases in these metabolites were not different by race. (From Brazerol et al., ref. 7, with permission.)

human skin. Matsuoka et al. (4) recently published a paper confirming that in the northern United States, winter UVB irradiance does not reach the threshold required for cutaneous synthesis of vitamin D$_3$, leaving individuals who live at northern latitudes highly dependent on body stores and dietary supply to meet vitamin D requirements during winter.

Atmospheric pollution may also increase atmospheric absorption and scattering of UVB, and could play an important role in some areas of the globe. The large epidemic of rickets that occurred at the beginning of industrialization occurred mostly in the major cities, where atmospheric pollution was considerable (5).

Exposure time to ultraviolet B, *skin surface area* exposed, and *skin pigmentation* may all play a significant role as well (1,6,7).

In a study by Brazerol et al. (7), black and white subjects were repeatedly exposed to a minimal erythematous dose of UVB over a period of 6 weeks. The rate of rise in serum 25-hydroxyvitamin D (25-OHD) or 24,25-dihydroxyvitamin D [24,25(OH)$_2$D] was similar in blacks and whites, although at baseline, black subjects had significantly lower values than white subjects (Fig. 1). However, Hollick et al. (1) showed that as skin pigmentation increases from type III (hypopigmented) to types V and VI (hyperpigmented), the time of a single exposure to UVB that is necessary to maximize previtamin D$_3$ formation increases from 30 minutes to 1 and 3 hours, respectively. Thus, the capacity to produce vitamin D in response to high ultraviolet B exposure seems to be the same in heavily pigmented individuals as in lightly pigmented individuals; however, heavy skin pigmentation theoretically may

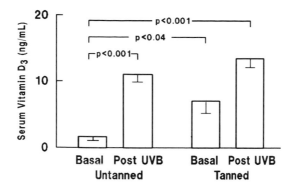

FIG. 2. Serum vitamin D_3 levels in seven healthy subjects. Determinations were performed during midwinter (*Untanned*) and midsummer (*Tanned*). On each occasion, blood was obtained before and 24 hours after whole-body exposure to a fixed dose of ultraviolet B (*UVB*) rays in a phototherapy unit. Tanning produces higher vitamin D_3 concentrations and attenuation of the response to UVB. (From Matsuoka et al., ref. 8, with permission.)

become a significant limiting factor in vitamin D production when exposure to UVB is borderline. Similarly, *skin tanning* also limits vitamin D production; as shown by Matsuoka and collaborators (8), tanned subjects will have a lesser increase in serum vitamin D_3 when they are exposed to UVB compared with the same subjects when untanned (Fig. 2). Evidently vitamin D status will be affected not only by vitamin D skin production, but also by dietary habits, as exogenous vitamin D might be a considerable source.

Vitamin D as a Prohormone

Vitamin D originates from skin (vitamin D_3 or cholecalciferol) or from exogenous dietary sources (vitamin D_2 or ergocalciferol from plant sources and vitamin D_3 from animal sources). In either instance, for maximum potency, vitamin D must be hydroxylated in the *liver* at the carbon 25 to form 25-OHD and then in the *kidney* at the carbon 1 to form 1,25-dihydroxyvitamin D [1,25(OH)$_2$D] (9). Dietary control, through a direct effect from serum calcium and serum phosphate concentrations, and hormonal control, through the effects of parathyroid hormone and possibly growth hormone and insulin, affect 1,25(OH)$_2$D production in the kidney (9). The implication of these successive hydroxylations is that in liver and renal failure, vitamin D requirements may be increased (9–11). In addition, since dietary vitamin D is absorbed in the intestine together with fats, it requires bile salts for micelle formation (10). In *cholestasis,* when bile salt secretion is impaired or absent, there is a potential for vitamin D malabsorption (10). Furthermore, vitamin D catabolism involves the cytochrome p 450 system in the liver. Since this system is activated by anticonvulsants such as phenobarbital or dilantin, the vitamin D half-life is reduced in patients receiving these drugs (12). Consequently, neonates born to mothers re-

ceiving anticonvulsants and infants receiving these drugs are at increased risk for
vitamin D deficiency (13).

Vitamin D Effects on Mineral Metabolism

Due to its combined effect in stimulating intestinal calcium absorption (14–16) and
bone resorption (17,18) (and possibly tubular reabsorption of filtered calcium in the
kidney), $1,25(OH)_2D$ has a potent hypercalcemic effect (19). It also increases phosphorus absorption in the intestine (19).

In spite of abundant research in the past century, the vitamin D effects on target
cells are still not completely clear (19). Like other steroid hormones, $1,25(OH)_2D$
binds to an intracellular receptor protein that translocates it to the cell nucleus.
Subsequently, messenger RNAs are induced that lead to the synthesis of specific
proteins such as calcium-binding protein. It remains unclear as to whether
$1,25(OH)_2D$ has a *direct action* on bone formation (20–25). However, there is indirect
evidence that there are $1,25(OH)_2D$ receptors on bone cells; also, synthesis of alkaline phosphatase and osteocalcin (both produced by osteoblasts, the bone-forming
cells) is stimulated by $1,25(OH)_2D$ (19). However, many investigators think that
vitamin D affects bone mineralization mostly by regulating calcium and phosphorus
transport, in order to maintain normal serum calcium and phosphorus concentration.

Consequences of Vitamin D Deficiency

In the absence of vitamin D, absorption of dietary calcium and phosphorus is not
maximized. As a consequence of, and to prevent a further drop in serum calcium
concentration, *secondary hyperparathyroidism* develops (26), which will correct hypocalcemia at the expense of bone calcium through bone resorption. Hyperparathyroidism aggravates urinary phosphate losses. Resulting hypophosphatemia will
lead to formation of unmineralized cartilage and bone matrix (27). In the most severe
stages, hypocalcemia may develop in spite of compensatory hyperparathyroidism,
leading to *hypocalcemic tetany* (28). Moreover, because normal local calcium concentration at the growth plate is necessary for chondroclast maturation, the cartilage
matrix is not resorbed. The width of the growth plates becomes enlarged, leading
to typical rachitic bone features. In addition, the hypophosphatemia often observed
in rickets may contribute to severe *muscle weakness* and generalized hypotonia.

Mize and collaborators used nuclear magnetic resonance to measure the ratio of
phosphocreatine/adenosine triphosphate (ATP) in skeletal muscle in vitamin D-dependent rickets (Fig. 3) (29). The increase of this ratio during therapy and its very
low level at baseline indicates that there was a relative cellular deficit in high-energy
phosphate-related metabolites in skeletal muscle, which was probably responsible
for the severe hypotonia in the patient studied (29).

In full-blown rickets, the classic clinical features include *craniotabes* ("ping-pong"
ball feeling upon pressure on the cranial bones, particularly in the occipital area);

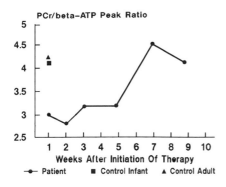

FIG. 3. Ratio of peak areas of phosphocreatine (*PCr*) to β-ATP in gastrocnemius of patient with vitamin D-dependent rickets (●) as a function of time after initiation of therapy. Control infants (age 6 months) and adult forearm peak ratios are indicated as ■ and ▲, respectively. (From Mize et al., ref. 29, with permission.)

rachitic *rosary* (enlargement of the chondrocostal junction); metaphysial enlargement at the wrists and ankles; deformities of spine, pelvis, and legs; ligamental laxity; and delayed dentition or delayed closure of the cranial sutures (27).

The x-rays shown in Fig. 4 are typical of rickets. There is a marked curvature of the long bones, the distal end appears widened, concave ("cupping"), and frayed, in contrast to the normal sharply demarcated and slightly convex ends, and the density of the shafts is decreased.

Other Functions of Vitamin D

Other functions of vitamin D are less understood, but may be of fundamental biologic importance. In the past few years, $1,25(OH)_2D$ has been shown to influence

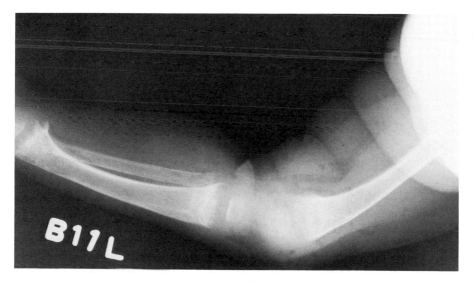

FIG. 4. Lower limb x-rays of a patient with vitamin D-deficient rickets. There is a marked curvature of the long bones; the distal end appears widened, concave (cupping), and frayed, in contrast to the normal sharply demarcated and slightly convex ends. The density of bone shafts is decreased.

cell proliferation and differentiation in several tissues and to have immunoregulatory properties (30–40). In the hemopoietic system, including lymphocytes and in many cancer cell systems, $1,25(OH)_2D$ has antiproliferative and differentiation-inducing effects. In cancer research, attempts are being made to develop vitamin D analogs that would keep the antiproliferative actions of the hormone without causing hypercalcemia (40). An antiproliferative effect of $1,25(OH)_2D$ on epidermal cells has also been described. This effect has been utilized in several clinical trials of psoriasis therapy (41,42).

VITAMIN D DEFICIENCY RICKETS IN THE WORLD

Bedouins Living in the Middle East

In Bedouin populations there is a lack of exposure to sunlight, probably for cultural reasons. These Muslim women cover most of their skin, including their face, leading to extraordinarily low concentrations of vitamin D in their blood and that of their infants in spite of the considerable potential for sunlight exposure in these areas. In addition, traditional Bedouin foods are not fortified with vitamin D (43,44).

Subcontinent Asians in Great Britain

Indian subcontinent Asians living in Great Britain have been studied extensively because of a high incidence of infantile rickets (45–50). In these patients and their parents, there is a combination of relatively darker skin pigmentation along with the atmospheric pollution of industrialized cities, vegetarianism, and a high intake of chupatty (a bread that contains calcium binders). The relative contribution of all these factors is still unclear. Nevertheless, infants born to Indian subcontinent Asians in Great Britain have lower vitamin D status at birth than British infants, and have higher serum parathyroid hormone concentrations, supporting the hypothesis of a possible functional hyperparathyroidism *in utero* (48,49).

Eskimos

In Eskimos, the relative lack of sunlight during the long arctic winter may play a predominant role in development of rickets (51); however, maternal mineral status might also be impaired by low calcium and high phosphorus intake, in that the traditional Eskimo diet consists primarily of meat.

Chinese Infants

Ten to twenty percent of breast-fed Chinese infants may have vitamin D deficiency, and up to 50% of the latter group may have rickets (52,53). Maternal vitamin

D status is often borderline, in that food in China is not vitamin D-fortified, making endogenous skin production the major source. However, other factors such as dietary calcium and phosphorus may be involved, since not all rachitic Chinese infants are vitamin D-deficient.

Black Breast-Fed Infants in the United States

Vitamin D deficiency in the United States is almost exclusively found in black breast-fed infants without vitamin D supplementation. Reports by Edidin in 1980 (54), Venkataraman in 1983 (26), or Kriegcr in 1985 (55), as well as our own experience, all confirm this finding. Similarly, a recent study of rachitic children in France reported that most patients were of African origin (56). Most cases are diagnosed between February and May. Rare additional cases are described in vegetarian families whose infants are not provided with any dairy or egg products (57).

To explain the susceptibility of black breast-fed infants to vitamin D deficiency or rickets requires a description of the vitamin D content of human milk. The major vitamin D metabolites present in human milk are vitamin D and 25-OHD, with minimal amounts of dihydroxylated metabolites (58,59). A water-soluble fraction, or vitamin D sulfate, has been identified, but its biological activity seems to be very low and its presence in human milk has been challenged (58). The total vitamin D and 25-OHD activity in human milk equals approximately 12–60 IU/l, far below the 400 IU/l present in fortified formulas (58).

Maternal vitamin D status seems to be the major factor regulating the vitamin D content of human milk; it is mostly influenced by maternal dietary vitamin D, sun exposure, and race.

Specker and collaborators (60) showed that breast milk vitamin D concentration correlates with maternal vitamin D intake (Fig. 4). Also, as shown by Greer et al. (61), there are very high concentrations of vitamin D_2 in the milk of mothers taking pharmacologic doses of vitamin D_2.

In another study, Greer et al. (62) administered UVB irradiation to lactating mothers: serum vitamin D_3 increased to reach a peak at 2 days postirradiation. Breast milk vitamin D content peaked 1 day later than the peak in serum, supporting the thesis that UVB irradiation can affect breast milk vitamin D_3 content.

In the United States, the vitamin D_3, D_2, 25-OHD_3, and 1,25$(OH)_2D$ content of the breast milk of black women was found to be lower than that of white women (60). Also, infant vitamin D status (assessed by 25-OHD concentration at birth) correlated strongly with that of the mother at the time of delivery (63–65). After birth, however, serum 25-OHD concentration strongly correlated with the infant's sun exposure (65).

Specker et al. (65) showed that serum 25-OHD follows a cyclical pattern during the year paralleling the cycle of seasonal sun exposure. In infants born in summer, serum 25-OHD concentrations dropped during the first 6 months of life (that is, in winter) and increased in the following 6 months; the opposite was true for infants born in winter. When sunshine exposure is expressed as a score or in minutes out-doors per day, the same cyclical variations occur, with an increase by age 6 months in sunshine exposure babies born in winter and a decrease by 6 months of age in babies born in summer (65). When the UV exposure score is extrapolated to minutes of exposure per week with reference to facial exposure only, it correlates strongly with infant 25-OHD concentration. Thus it is believed that the breast-fed infant is generally dependent on sunshine exposure to achieve adequate vitamin D status (65). However, in periods of inadequate sunshine exposure, the (relatively low) vitamin D concentrations of human milk might become significant.

CURRENT RDAS VERSUS REAL LIFE

RDAs for Formula-Fed Infants

The current vitamin D RDAs (based on limited data) are 300 IU/day before the age of 6 months and 400 IU/day for the remainder of the first year of life (66). At this level of intake, there have been no reports of vitamin D deficiency rickets. Healthy formula-fed infants consume approximately 700–800 ml of formula per day between the ages of 16 and 26 weeks of life (67). Thus their vitamin D intake is approximately 300 IU/day, which corresponds exactly to the RDA. However, *de-creased* or *increased* formula intake has the potential of significantly modifying vi-tamin D intake. Furthermore, 300–400 IU/day might still be in excess of that nec-essary to prevent rickets. As an example, in a study of 256 Chinese infants in China randomized to 50, 100, or 200 IU vitamin D per day, none of the infants showed radiological signs of rickets at 6 months of age (Dr. B. Specker, personal commu-nication). The issue of vitamin D toxicity is not resolved, as a daily dose at which toxicity can be predicted is unknown. In one study, daily intake of 1,800–6,300 IU inhibited linear growth in normal infants (68). Toxicity at lower doses has not been clearly identified. Thus it appears that the RDAs may have been set at an excessive, but apparently safe level.

RDAs for Breast-Fed Infants

Supplementation for breast-fed infants is a more complex issue. The current RDA reads as follows: "Breast-fed infants who are not exposed to sunlight should receive a daily supplement of 200–300 IU of vitamin D (66). There are no recommendations for breast-fed infants who are exposed to sunlight, nor are the RDAs differentiated by race. From available evidence, it appears that the black breast-fed infant *should* receive vitamin D supplements at least throughout winter. The issue of white breast-fed infants is more controversial: theoretically, in Cincinnati, Ohio, being outdoors for 30 minutes a week fully clothed without a hat should be sufficient to maintain an adequate vitamin D status (65). However, this kind of exposure might not be sufficient in other areas in the United States.

In a study conducted in Cincinnati by Greer et al. (69), breast-fed infants were randomized to receive vitamin D supplementation (400 IU/day) or placebo. Infants in the vitamin D group had a higher bone mineral content (similar to formula-fed infants) at 12 weeks of age than those who received placebo. They also had a higher serum 25-OHD concentration. The placebo group had a mean 25-OHD concentration below 10 ng/ml at 26 weeks (considered to be in the rachitic range). No x-rays were taken to confirm or rule out rickets in these patients. The difference in bone mineral content between the two breast-fed groups disappeared by 26 weeks of age. A similar study conducted by the same primary investigator in Madison, Wisconsin (70) failed to reproduce these differences. In this report, patients who received vitamin D_2 as a supplement had a significant increase in 25-OHD_2 over time. The group on formula (formulas are fortified with vitamin D_3) and the breast-fed group without D_2 supplements, as expected, had low serum 25-OHD_2 concentrations. Serum 25-OHD_3 rose significantly in the formula group and stayed higher than in the two breast milk groups. Surprisingly, bone mineral content was not higher at 3 months or 6 months of age in the vitamin D-supplemented breast-fed group, compared with the breast-fed group that was not supplemented. Bone mineral content was higher in the formula group than in the breast-fed groups, confirming previous findings. No x-ray was obtained to confirm or rule out rickets.

A study was done of breast-fed infants born in the Netherlands at the end of summer who had a high vitamin D status at birth. By 8 weeks of age, 70 percent had a plasma 25-OHD concentration below the fifth adult reference percentile (71). The authors of this report concluded that vitamin D stores at birth were depleted after 8 weeks of winter.

In a study conducted in Finland (72), maternal supplementation at 1,000 IU/day did not prevent the infant's serum 25-OHD concentrations from dropping rapidly to less than 5 ng/ml (an extremely low level) in 10 of 18 breast-fed unsupplemented infants.

Vitamin D supplementation practices for breast-fed infants were studied recently by Hayward and collaborators (73); these authors showed that length of practice in pediatrics significantly affected the use of multivitamins: 55% of pediatricians in practice for less than 10 years prescribed vitamin D supplementation for breast-fed infants, while 84% in practice for more than 10 years prescribed vitamin D for breast-fed infants; thus the use of vitamin D in breast-fed infants appears to be less "fashionable" among younger pediatricians.

Use of Sunscreens

The use of sunscreens may create a new problem. Indeed, due to public awareness of the relationship between sunlight exposure and skin cancer, sunscreens are used increasingly in the United States in summer (74). Sunscreens recommended by manufacturers for infants are extremely efficient and completely or almost completely block UVB photons. Growing use of sunscreens might lead in the future to a modification of the RDAs, as infants born at the start of summer may not be able to "store" sufficient amounts for the winter.

CONCLUSIONS

At the present time, RDAs for vitamin D are more than adequate. The question of whether breast-fed infants should or should not be supplemented with vitamin D cannot be answered at the present time. Large studies involving x-ray diagnosis of rickets are required. These studies should be conducted at various latitudes and seasons, and should take into account the infant's skin pigmentation and sun exposure practices. However, it seems prudent to supplement at least all black breast-fed infants in winter, regardless of the latitude, as nutritional rickets in these infants has been described in latitudes as southern as San Diego, California.

ACKNOWLEDGMENTS

This work was supported in part by NIH grants HD-11725, RR-00068, and HD-20748, and a grant from the 25-Club, Magee-Womens Hospital.

REFERENCES

1. Holick MF. The cutaneous photosynthesis of previtamin D_3: a unique photoendocrine system. *J Invest Dermatol* 1981;76:51–58.
2. Webb AR, Kline L, Holick MF. Influence of season and latitude on the cutaneous synthesis of vitamin D_3: exposure to winter sunlight in Boston and Edmonton will not promote vitamin D_3 synthesis in human skin. *J Clin Endocrinol Metab* 1988;67:373–378.
3. McLaughlin M, Fairney A, Lester E, Raggatt PR, Brown DJ, Wills MR. Seasonal variations in serum 25-hydroxycholecalciferol in healthy people. *Lancet* 1974;i:536–538.
4. Matsuoka LY, Wortsman J, Haddad JG, Hollis BW. In vivo threshold for cutaneous synthesis of vitamin D_3. *J Lab Clin Med* 1989;114:301–305.
5. Harrison HE, Harrison HC. Rickets then and now. *J Pediatr* 1975;87:1144–1151.
6. Clemens TL, Adams JS, Henderson SL, Holick MF. Increased skin pigment reduces the capacity of skin to synthesise vitamin D_3. *Lancet* 1982;75–76.
7. Brazerol WF, McPhee AJ, Mimouni F, Specker BL, Tsang RC. Serial ultraviolet B exposure and serum 25 hydroxyvitamin D response in young adult American blacks and whites: no racial differences. *Am J Coll Nutr* 1988;7:111–118.
8. Matsuoka LY, Wortsman J, Hollis BW. Suntanning and cutaneous synthesis of vitamin D_3. *J Lab Clin Med* 1990;116:87–90.
9. Rosen JF, Chesney RW. Circulating calcitriol concentrations in health and disease. *J Pediatr* 1983;103:1–17.
10. Heubi JE, Hollis BW, Specker B, Tsang RC. Bone disease in chronic childhood cholestasis. I. Vitamin D absorption and metabolism. *Hepatology* 1989;9:258–264.
11. Nordal KP, Dahl E. Low dose calcitriol versus placebo in patients with predialysis chronic renal failure. *J Clin Endocrinol Metab* 1988;67:929–936.
12. Hahn TJ, Birge SJ, Scharp CR, Avioli LV. Phenobarbital-induced alterations in vitamin D metabolism. *J Clin Invest* 1972;51:741–748.
13. Markestad T, Ulstein M, Strandjord RE, Aksnes L, Aarskog D. Anticonvulsant drug therapy in human pregnancy: effects on serum concentrations of vitamin D metabolites in maternal and cord blood. *Am J Obstet Gynecol* 1984;150:254–258.

14. Nemere I, Norman AW. 1,25-dihydroxyvitamin D_3-mediated vesicular transport of calcium in intestine: time course studies. *Endocrinology* 1988;122:2962–2969.

15. Ghishan FK, Leonard D, Pietsch J. Calcium transport by plasma membranes of enterocytes during development: role of 1,25 $(OH)_2$ vitamin D_3. *Pediatr Res* 1988;24:338–341.

16. Thomasset M, Cuisinier-Gleizes P, Mathieu H. 1,25 dihydroxycalciferol: dynamics of the stimulation of duodenal calcium-binding protein, calcium transport, and bone calcium mobilization in vitamin D and calcium-deficient rats. *FEBS Lett* 1979;107:91–94.

17. Weisbrode SE, Capen CC, Norman AW. Ultrastructural evaluation of the effects of 1,25-dihydroxyvitamin D_3 on bone of thyroparathyroidectomized rats fed a low-calcium diet. *Am J Pathol* 1978;92:459–465.

18. Brommage R, Neuman WF. Mechanism of mobilization of bone mineral by 1,25-dihydroxyvitamin D_3. *Am J Physiol* 1979;237:E113–E120.

19. Reichel H, Koeffler HP, Norman AW. The role of the vitamin D endocrine system in health and disease. *N Engl J Med* 1989;320:980–991.

20. Underwood JL, DeLuca HF. Vitamin D is not directly necessary for bone growth and mineralization. *Am J Physiol* 1984;246:E493–E498.

21. Norman AW, Leathers V, Bishop JE. Normal egg hatchability requires the simultaneous administration of the hen of 1α, 25-dihydroxycholecalciferol and 24R, 25-dihydroxycholecalciferol. *J Nutr* 1983;113:2505–2515.

22. Boyan BD, Schwartz Z, Carnes DL, Ramirez V. The effects of vitamin D metabolites on the plasma and matrix vesicle membranes of growth and resting cartilage cells in vitro. *Endocrinology* 1988;122:2851–2860.

23. Gerstenfeld LC, Kelly CM, Von Deck M, Lian JB. Effect of 1,25-dihydroxyvitamin D_3 on induction of chondrocyte maturation in culture: extracellular matrix gene expression and morphology. *Endocrinology* 1990;126:1599–1609.

24. Parfitt AM, Mathews CHE, Brommage R, Jarnagin K, DeLuca HF. Calcitriol but no other metabolite of vitamin D is essential for normal bone growth and development in the rat. *J Clin Invest* 1984;73:576–586.

25. Brommage R, DeLuca HF. Evidence that 1,25-dihydroxyvitamin D_3 is the physiologically active metabolite of vitamin D_3. *Endocrinol Rev* 1985;6:491–511.

26. Venkataraman PS, Tsang RC, Buckley DD, Ho M, Steichen JJ. Elevation of serum 1,25-dihydroxyvitamin D in response to physiologic doses of vitamin D in vitamin D-deficient infants. *J Pediatr* 1983;103:416–419.

27. Barness LA. Rickets of vitamin D deficiency. In: Berhman RE, Vaughan III VC, Nelson NE, eds. *Nelson textbook of pediatrics*, 12th ed. Philadelphia: WB Saunders Company, 1983;179–183.

28. Barness LA. Tetany of vitamin D deficiency. In: Berhman RE, Vaughan III VC, Nelson NE, eds. *Nelson textbook of pediatrics*, 12th ed. Philadelphia: WB Saunders Company, 1983;183–184.

29. Mize CE, Corbett RJT, Uauy R, Nunnally RL, Williamson SB. Hypotonia of rickets: a sequential study by P-31 magnetic resonance spectroscopy. *Pediatr* Res 1988;24:713–716.

30. Bar Shavit Z, Noff D, Edelstein S, Meyer M, Shibolet S, Goldman R. 1,25 dihydroxyvitamin D_3 and the regulation of macrophage function. *Calcif Tissue Int* 1981;33:673–676.

31. Abe E, Miyaura C, Sakagami H, et al. Differentiation of mouse myeloid leukemia cells induced by 1α 25-dihydroxyvitamin D_3. *Proc Natl Acad Sci USA* 1981;78:4990–4904.

32. Bar-Shavit Z, Teitelbaum SL, Reitsma P, et al. Induction of monocytic differentiation and bone resorption by a 1,25-dihydroxyvitamin D_3. *Proc Natl Acad Sci USA* 1983;80:5907–5911.

33. McCarthy DM, San Miguel JF, Freake HC, et al. 1,25-dihydroxyvitamin D_3 inhibits proliferation of human promyelocytic leukaemia (HL60) cells and induces monocyte-macrophage differentiation in HL60 and normal human bone marrow cells. *Leuk Res* 1983;7:51–55.

34. Mangelsdorf DJ, Koeffler HP, Donaldson CA, Pike JW, Haussler MR. 1,25-Dihydroxyvitamin D_3-induced differentiation in a human promyelocytic leukemia cell line (HL-60): receptor-mediated maturation to macrophage-like cells. *J Cell Biol* 1984;98:391–398.

35. Tsoukas CD, Provvedini DM, Manolagas SC. 1,25-dihydroxyvitamin D_3: a novel immunoregulatory hormone. *Science* 1984;224:1438–1440.

36. Iho S, Takahashi T, Kura F, Sugiyama H, Hoshino T. The effect of 1,25-dihydroxyvitamin D_3 on in vitro immunoglobulin production in human B cells. *J Immunol* 1986;136:4427–4431.

37. Lemire JM, Adams JS, Kermani-Arab V, Bakke AC, Sakai R, Jordan SC. 1,25-Dihydroxyvitamin D_3 suppresses human T helper/inducer lymphocyte activity in vitro. *J Immunol* 1985;134:3032–3035.

38. Fujita T, Matsui T, Nakao Y, Watanabe S. T lymphocyte subsets in osteoporosis. Effect of 1-alpha hydroxyvitamin D_3. *Miner Electrolyte Metab* 1984;10:375–378.

39. Frampton RJ, Omond SA, Eisman JA. Inhibition of human cancer cell growth by 1,25-dihydroxy-vitamin D₃ metabolites. *Cancer Res* 1983;43:4443–4447.
40. Abe J, Takita Y, Nakano T, Miyaura C, Suda T, Nishii Y. A synthetic analogue of vitamin D₃, 22-oxa-1α, 25-dihydroxyvitamin D₃, is a potent modulator of in vivo immunoregulating activity without inducing hypercalcemia in mice. *Endocrinology* 1989;124:2645–2647.
41. Kuroki T. Possible functions of 1α, 25-dihydroxyvitamin D₃, an active form of vitamin D₃, in the differentiation and development of skin. *J Invest Dermatol* 1985;84:459–460.
42. Abe J, Kondo S, Nishii Y, Kuroki T. Resistance to 1,25-dihydroxyvitamin D₃ of cultured psoriatic epidermal keratinocytes isolated from involved and uninvolved skin. *J Clin Endocrinol Metab* 1989;68:851–854.
43. Taha SA, Dost SM, Sedrani SH. 25-Hydroxyvitamin D and total calcium: extraordinarily low plasma concentrations in Saudi mothers and their neonates. *Pediatr Res* 1984;18:739–741.
44. Shany S, Biale Y, Zuili I, Yankowitz N, Berry JL, Mawer EB. Feto-maternal relationships between vitamin D metabolites in Israeli Bedouins and Jews. *Am J Clin Nutr* 1984;40:1290–1294.
45. Watney PJM, Chance GW, Scott P, Thompson JM. Maternal factors in neonatal hypocalcemia. A study in three ethnic groups. *Br Med J* 1971;2:432–436.
46. Preece MA, McIntosh WB, Tomlinson S, Ford JA, Dunnigan MG, O'Riordan JLH. Vitamin-D deficiency among Asian immigrants to Britain. *Lancet* 1973;i:907–910.
47. Robinson D, Flynn D, Dandona P. Hyperphosphataemic rickets in an Asian infant. *Br Med J* 1985;290:1318–1319.
48. Okonofua F, Menon RK, Houlder S, et al. Parathyroid hormone and neonatal calcium homeostasis: evidence for secondary hyperparathyroidism in the Asian neonate. *Metabolism* 1986;35:803–806.
49. Okonofua F, Menon RK, Houlder S, et al. Calcium, vitamin D and parathyroid hormone relationships in pregnant Caucasian and Asian women and their neonates. *Ann Clin Biochem* 1987;24:22–28.
50. Henderson JB, Dunnigan MG, McIntosh WB, Abdul-Motaal AA, Gettinby G, Glekin BM. The importance of limited exposure to ultraviolet radiation and dietary factors in the aetiology of Asian rickets: a risk-factor model. *Q J Med* 1987;63:413–425.
51. Mazess RB, Barden HS, Christiansen C, Harper AB, Laughlin WS. Bone mineral and vitamin D in Aleutian Islanders. *Am J Clin Nutr* 1985;42:143–146.
52. Xiao L. Survey on infant rickets. *J Chinese Pediatr* (in Chinese) 1982;20:63–70.
53. Ho ML, Yen HC, Tsang RC, Specker BL, Chen XC, Nichols BL. Randomized study of sunshine exposure and serum 25-OHD in breast-fed infants in Beijing, China. *J Pediatr* 1985;107:928–931.
54. Edidin DV, Leritsky L, Schey W, et al. Resurgence of nutritional rickets associated with breast feeding and special dietary practices. *Pediatrics* 1980;65:232–235.
55. Krieger I. Nutritional rickets returns. *Pediatr Consult* Fall 1985:113–114.
56. Garabedian M, Vainsel M, Mallet E, et al. Circulating vitamin D metabolite concentrations in children with nutritional rickets. *J Pediatr* 1983;103:381–386.
57. Hellebostad M, Markestad T, Seeger Halvorsen K. Vitamin D deficiency rickets and vitamin B₁₂ deficiency in vegetarian children. *Acta Paediatr Scand* 1985;74:191–195.
58. Makin HLJ, Seamark DA, Trafford DJH. Vitamin D and its metabolites in human breast milk. *Arch Dis Child* 1983;58:750–753.
59. Ballester I, Cortes E, Moya M, Campello MJ. Improved method for quantifying vitamin D in proprietary infants' formulas and in breast milk. *Clin Chem* 1987;33:796–799.
60. Specker BL, Tsang RC, Hollis BW. Effect of race and diet on human-milk vitamin D and 25-hydroxyvitamin D. *Am J Dis Child* 1985;139:1134–1137.
61. Greer FR, Hollis BW, Napoli JL. High concentrations of vitamin D₂ in human milk associated with pharmacologic doses of vitamin D₂. *J Pediatr* 1984;105:61–64.
62. Greer FR, Hollis BW, Cripps DJ, Tsang RC. Effects of maternal ultraviolet B irradiation on vitamin D content of human milk. *J Pediatr* 1984;105:431–433.
63. Specker BL, Valanis B, Hertzberg V, Edwards N, Tsang RC. Sunshine exposure and serum 25-hydroxyvitamin D concentrations in exclusively breast-fed infants. *J Pediatr* 1985;107:372–376.
64. Specker BL, Tsang RC, Ho M, Buckley D. Seasonal differences in serum vitamin D binding protein in exclusively breast-fed infants: negative relationship to sunshine exposure and 25-hydroxyvitamin D. *J Pediatr Gastroenterol Nutr* 1986;5:290–294.
65. Specker BL, Tsang RC. Cyclical serum 25-hydroxyvitamin D₃ concentrations paralleling sunshine exposure in exclusively breast-fed infants. *J Pediatr* 1987;110:744–747.
66. Subcommittee on the Tenth Edition of the RDAs. Vitamin D. In: *Recommended dietary allowances,* 10th ed. Washington, DC: National Academy Press, 1989;92–98.

67. Kohler L, Meeuwisse G, Mortensson W. Food intake and growth of infants between six and twenty-six weeks of age on breast milk, cow's milk formula, or soy formula. *Acta Paediatr Scand* 1984;73:40–48.
68. AAP (American Academy of Pediatrics): The prophylactic requirement and the toxicity of vitamin D. *Pediatrics* 1963;31:512–525.
69. Greer FR, Searcy JF, Levin RS, Steichen JJ, Steichen-Asche PS, Tsang RC. Bone mineral content and serum 25-hydroxyvitamin D concentrations in breast-fed infants with and without supplemental Vitamin D: one-year follow-up. *J Pediatr* 1982;100:919–922.
70. Greer FR, Marshall S. Bone mineral content, serum vitamin D metabolite concentrations, and ultraviolet B light exposure in infants fed human milk with and without vitamin D_2 supplements. *J Pediatr* 1989;114:204–212.
71. Hoogenboezem T, Degenhart HJ, de Muinck Keizer-Schrama SMPF, et al. Vitamin D metabolism in breast-fed infants and their mothers. *Pediatr Res* 1989;25:623–628.
72. Ala-Houhala M. 25-Hydroxyvitamin D levels during breast-feeding with or without maternal or infantile supplementation of vitamin D. *J Pediatr Gastroenterol Nutr* 1985;4:220–226.
73. Hayward I, Stein MT, Gibson MI. Nutritional rickets in San Diego. *Am J Dis Child* 1987;141:1060–1062.
74. National Institutes of Health Consensus Development Conference Statement: Sunlight, ultraviolet radiation and the skin. NIH publication, vol 7, no 8. Washington, DC: US Government Printing Office, 1989;1–10.

Calcium Nutriture for Mothers and Children, edited by
Reginald C. Tsang and Francis Mimouni. Carnation
Nutrition Education Series, Vol. 3. Carnation Co.,
Glendale/Raven Press, Ltd., New York © 1992.

The Osteoporotic Problem

Louis V. Avioli

*Division of Bone and Mineral Diseases, Washington University School of Medicine;
and Section of Endocrinology and Metabolism, The Jewish Hospital of St. Louis,
St. Louis, Missouri 63110*

Osteoporosis is a metabolic bone disease in which the amount of normally mineralized bone has been reduced to a level where the risk of fractures occurring in the absence of trauma or in response to trivial trauma (fall from a standing height or less) is increased, or such fractures have already occurred. Some authorities distinguish osteoporosis without fracture from osteoporosis with fracture by using the term *osteopenia* for the former condition and restricting the use of the term *osteoporosis* to patients who have already sustained a nontraumatic vertebral fracture. Thus the relationship between osteopenia and osteoporosis would be similar to the relationship between hypertension and stroke. This analogy can lead to quantitative definitions of osteopenia and osteoporosis, which are gaining wider acceptance. Osteopenia can be defined as a reduction in bone mass to below peak adult bone mass or a reduction in bone mass to below the theoretical fracture threshold. An additional important aspect of any definition of osteoporosis is the concept that the amount of bone is reduced although the mineral–collagen ratio is normal. Thus osteoporosis can be distinguished from osteomalacia, a bone disease that may present with either normal, decreased, or increased bone mass although the tissue is always relatively deficient in mineral (1).

EPIDEMIOLOGY

Osteoporosis is the most prevalent metabolic bone disease in Western societies where nutrition is adequate, although on a world-wide basis rickets and osteomalacia secondary to nutritional deficiency of vitamin D and limited exposure to sunlight is probably more prevalent. Women with the lowest peak adult bone mass have the highest prevalence of osteoporosis. With 25–35 million American women suffering from osteoporosis, the disease is as common as hypertension and more common than diabetes, breast cancer, alcoholism, and arthritis (2,3). In fact, results of the U.S. HANES I study reveal that any estimated incidence of osteopenia may reflect the "tip of the iceberg" since it fails to account for the subtle abnormal loss of bone mass in premenopausal women that was determined in the HANES I study to exist in 6–8 percent of women between 25 and 34 years of age (4). It has been estimated that 30 percent of all postmenopausal white women sustain at least one osteoporotic fracture during life, and the incidence increases with advancing age. Black individuals, who characteristically acquire a peak adult bone mass much greater than that of nonblack populations, rarely sustain atraumatic osteoporotic fractures.

Vertebral fractures, which are much more common in women than in men, may occur before the clinical menopause due to asymptomatic disturbances in ovulation or gradual loss of ovarian function (5,6). Current statistics regarding the true incidence of nontraumatic vertebral fractures in postmenopausal women are fraught with interpretative difficulties, since *over 35% of vertebral fractures are silent*. The incidence of hip fractures in women actually begins to increase during the latter part of the fifth decade and increases progressively with age thereafter; women are affected two times more often than men (7). Up to 33 percent of women and more than 17 percent of men experience a hip fracture by age 90 years (2,3). Approximately 300,000 new cases of hip fractures resulting from osteoporosis occurred in 1989. This figure has been increasing for the last 10 years and is greater than expected from population growth statistics (2,3).

Several hypotheses have been put forward, the most logical of which is that age-related bone loss is a universal phenomenon in humans and that the increased prevalence of osteoporosis reflects a combination of an increase in the number of elderly as well as a variety of risk factors associated with daily living (1–3). The age-related decrease in both appendicular (long bones) and axial (spine) bone mass, which is accelerated in the immediate postmenopausal years, also continues after the seventh decade of life.

CLINICAL MANIFESTATIONS

Osteopenia defined only on the basis of a low bone mass (i.e., no fractures) is asymptomatic. The clinical hallmark of osteoporosis is fracture with associated pain and deformity. Many osteoporotic vertebral fractures are asymptomatic, however, presenting only with height loss or deformity, most commonly an increase in thoracic kyphosis ("dowager's hump"). The most common sites of fracture are distal radius (Colles' fracture), vertebral body, proximal femur, humerus, ribs, and distal femur (1). Osteoporotic long bone fractures respond well to standard conservative orthopedic treatment, with full recovery of shape and function the desired result. Fractures of the proximal femur (hip) are an important exception. Despite major improvements in surgical and anesthetic techniques, there is still a 15–20 percent mortality within the first 3 months following a hip fracture. Perhaps more importantly, the majority of patients who do survive this critical period rarely regain their prefracture functional state; approximately one-third of all hip fracture patients require some form of institutional care. Inadequate healing and chronic pain not infrequently result in increased psychological distress and greater functional impairment in the hip fracture patient (1). It is worth noting parenthetically that estimates of the health-care costs associated annually with osteoporosis, due primarily to the cost incurred by hip fractures, are escalating. The cost components of osteoporosis care for American women that were due primarily to the hip fracture "problem" approximated 5–6 billion dollars in 1986 (8). The breakdown was as follows: inpatient care: $2.8 billion; nursing home care, 2.1 billion; and outpatient care, $0.2 billion. These figures should increase progressively with time since, while the U.S. population has been increasing at an average annual rate of 1 percent, the Medicare (>65 years of age) population has been increasing at twice that rate (2.1 percent/year), and the age 85- or over subpopulation has been increasing at over four times that rate, at 4.6 percent/year (2,3).

Vertebral fractures heal well, but the shape deformity persists, so that chronic back pain, loss of height, increased kyphosis (thoracic vertebral fracture), decreased lumbar lordosis (lumbar vertebral fracture), and painful "low back pain" syndromes often due to pseudospondylolithesis are characteristic features of this syndrome. As height is lost progressively, the lower ribs approximate the pelvic brim, the abdomen becomes protuberant, and a variety of gastrointestinal complaints such as constipation and abdominal pain syndromes occur.

PATHOGENESIS

During childhood and adolescence bones not only grow in size, strength, and mineral content, but also change in composition and shape. The process(es) regulating the change in shape and composition is termed *bone modeling*. After puberty, when bone mass in boys and girls is similar (9), bone mineral content and bone strength continue to increase until the middle of the fourth decade (9,10). At that time bone mass in the upper extremities is greater in men than women, whereas no sex difference in bone mass occurs in the femoral neck region of the lower extremity, and vertebral bone mass is greater in females (10). After the adult "peak" bone mass has been attained, there is a progressive continual removal of old bone (bone resorption) and replacement (bone formation). This latter process, which is "coupled," is termed bone remodeling. Whereas 85–90 percent of bone mass accumulates before age 20 as the skeleton grows and is modeled, 10–15 percent of the total bone mass accumulates in the appendicular skeleton (i.e., long bones, comprised primarily of compact bone) during remodeling between ages 20–35 after cessation of statural growth when peak bone mass is established (10).

A variety of factors are essential to ensure the accumulation of a maximal amount of bone during periods of statural growth and bone modeling, not the least of which are familial and genetic influences and elemental calcium (11–13). Accumulated data also revealed that increased calcium supplementation in growing children may also prove beneficial to bone even when dietary calcium intake appears adequate. A variety of drugs (Table 1), if administered during the period of rapid skeletal growth, may also compromise maximal skeletal development of later years. This interference with the achievement of that maximal peak bone mass that might have been obtained in health also occurs when diseases complicate the pubescent period of life.

TABLE 1. *Factors commonly associated with osteopenic and/or osteoporotic syndrome*

Genetic
   White or Asiatic ethnicity
   Positive family history
   Small body frame (less than 127 lbs.)
Lifestyle
   Smoking
   Inactivity
   Nulliparity
   Excessive exercise (producing amenorrhea)
   Early natural menopause
   Late menarche
Nutritional factors
   Milk intolerance
   Life-long low dietary calcium intake
   Vegetarian diet
   Excessive alcohol intake
   Consistently high protein intake
Medical disorders
   Anorexia nervosa
   Thyrotoxicosis
   Parathyroid overactivity
   Cushing's syndrome
   Type I diabetes
   Alterations in gastrointestinal and hepatobiliary function
   Occult osteogenesis imperfecta
   Mastocytosis
   Rheumatoid arthritis
   "Transient" osteoporosis
   Prolonged parenteral nutrition
   Prolactinoma
   Hemolytic anemia
Drugs
   Thyroid replacement therapy
   Glucocorticoids
   Anticoagulants
   Chronic lithium therapy
   Chemotherapy (breast cancer or lymphoma)
   GnRH agonist or antagonist therapy
   Anticonvulsants
   Chronic phosphate binding antacid use
   Extended tetracycline use[a]
   Diuretics producing calciuria[a]
   Phenothiozine derivatives[a]
   Cyclosporin A

[a] Not yet associated with decreased bone mass in humans although identified as either toxic to bone in animals or as inducing calciuria and/or calcium malabsorption in humans.

TABLE 2. *Causes of osteoporosis in children*

"Transient osteoporosis"
Malabsorption syndromes
Chronic renal diseases
Chronic hepatobiliary disease
Chronic metabolic acidosis
Type I, diabetes
Cushing's syndrome
Inherited disorders
   Osteogenesis imperfecta
   Hypophosphatasia
   Homocystinuria
   Riley-Day syndrome
   Menkes' syndrome
   Ehlers-Danlos syndrome
   Lysinuric protein intolerance
Cystic fibrosis
Down's syndrome
Leukemias
Drug regimens
   Thyroid
   Glucocorticoid
   Immunosuppressive
   Anticonvulsant
Hypogonadism
   Kleinfelter's syndrome
   Turner's syndrome
Immobilization
Juvenile rheumatoid arthritis
Hyperparathyroidism
Hyperthyroidism
Vitamin C deficiency
Idiopathic scoliosis
Coeliac disease
Systemic lupus erythematosus
Inflammatory bowel disease
Total parenteral nutrition
Anorexia nervosa
Amenorrheic athletes (females)
Thalassemia
Chronic ethanol ingestion
? Constitutional delay in development

Decreased skeletal mass in children, observed before cessation of statural growth, is now a well-defined entity due primarily to the use of noninvasive methods of measuring quantitative bone mass such as dual-energy radiography and dual-photon densitometry (1). As noted in Table 2, the etiology of bone mass deficits observed during childhood and adolescent years encompasses a wide variety of disorders. This diverse spectrum results from either inherited defects in bone collagen and mineral profiles, alterations in the biological activation of vitamin D and circulating bone "growth factors," disorders in calcium absorption and/or excretion, and in some instances, adverse direct effects of drugs on bone cell function. Individuals with a propensity toward subtle losses in bone mass resulting from factor(s) listed in Table 2 should be subjected to noninvasive bone mass quantitation using commercially available procedures, which currently offer highly sensitive and precise measurements. Preventive programs should be established in those children with normal bone mass when risk factors for losing skeletal mass are anticipated (such as thyroid, glucocorticoid, immunosuppressive, and anticonvulsant therapies). Whenever practical and appropriate, therapeutic intervention (with predetermined serial bone mass measurement follow-up) should be considered when skeletal mass has already been compromised by risk factor(s) or disease processes.

Shortly after *peak adult bone mass* is attained in the fourth decade of life, a progressive net loss of bone ensues, the latter resulting from an imbalance between the bone formation and bone resorption "coupling" phenomenon. As noted earlier, this *age-related bone loss* is universal in humans. It has not yet been established with any certainty precisely when bone modeling ceases and bone remodeling begins or how this change is regulated. There is evidence that peak adult bone mass is attained at different times in men and in women (possibly also in blacks and in whites) and at different times in different bones or at least in different skeletal compartments (cortical and cancellous) (1). A variety of conditions and diseases result in *accelerated bone loss* so that a measurement of bone mass at any one time reflects peak adult bone mass *minus* any age-related bone loss. Thus, osteopenia or osteoporosis with fractures in later life will result from those diseases/conditions associated with poor bone growth and development and/or those conditions/diseases associated with accelerated bone loss (1). Those factors that predispose to an accelerated loss of bone during the aging process are also listed in Table 1. A low bone mass is the most important determinant of the risk of sustaining an osteoporotic fracture, but bone quality and also the risk of falling are important cofactors. Older people, in whom the prevalence of osteoporosis is greatest, are also more likely to fall as a result of failing vision and impaired neuromuscular coordination, and often because of medications that cause axial or postural hypotension (14–16).

CLINICAL EVALUATION

Bone mass can be reliably measured by a variety of noninvasive techniques such as single-photon densitometers, computed axial tomography (CAT) scanning, and dual-energy radiography (1). Standard radiographs are now considered too crude for reliable assessment of bone mass in the spine, but semiquantitative techniques such as metacarpal morphometry still have some value when the more modern and much more precise techniques are not available. Bone mass, however measured, should be related to normal values specific for the patient's gender and race. It should also be related to the patient's age and to the theoretical "fracture threshold" for the technique being used in order to establish the degree of osteopenia. Obviously the diagnosis of osteoporosis with fractures depends on an analysis of appropriate radiographs.

The next phase of the clinical evaluation is to ascertain whether the osteopenia/ osteoporosis is primary or secondary. Review of the causes of accelerated bone loss detailed in Table 1 should direct this evaluation both by careful history taking and physical examination and a few simple laboratory investigations. Most of the information can be gleaned from standard hematology and biochemistry profiles, which generally provide sufficient clues to potential alternative diagnoses such as osteomalacia, hyperparathyroidism, intestinal malabsorption, or chronic dilantin, glucocorticoid, or thyroid therapy. Since "thyroid excess" syndromes do result in more rapid bone loss, inappropriate use of thyroid hormone preparations should be curtailed, and subtle forms of hyperparathyroidism treated appropriately. Hyperparathyroidism is also a common endocrine disorder in the postmenopausal female; it may be subtle and is often masked, especially in patients on estrogen therapy. A high index of suspicion should also be maintained for multiple myeloma, since this disorder can result in significant generalized skeletal demineralization with or without fractures before other clinical features of the disease are manifest. Hyperglobulinemia or anemia may offer helpful clues for diagnosing multiple myeloma. Serum and urine protein electrophoresis should be performed, especially in anemic patients with high erythrocyte sedimentation rates (<30). On rare occasions, the diagnosis can only be made by bone marrow aspiration. In the presence of fracture and back pain, an in-depth pursuit of subtle forms of metastatic cancers (i.e., breast, stomach, lung, and uterus) is also advised since the unsuspecting elderly woman with osteopenia may also present with skeletal metastases. Hypogonadism is a frequent cause of osteoporosis in men, and recent therapeutic intervention for prostatic cancer with luteinizing hormone releasing hormone (LHRH) agonists or antagonists will predispose to more rapid bone loss. In addition to obtaining an adequate history for chronic alcoholism and/or immobilization and completing a thorough physical examination, measurement of gonadal function should be performed in all men with osteoporosis.

Typically, the standard biochemical tests of bone and mineral metabolism are normal in patients with age-related forms of osteoporosis, although circulating parathyroid hormone levels may be elevated in more elderly individuals with poor sunlight exposure and marginal intakes of calcium. Specifically, serum and urine calcium and inorganic phosphate are normal, as is the circulating alkaline phosphatase (although this latter may be elevated in patients with skeletal fractures). More specific biochemical markers of skeletal metabolism are available such as serum measurements of bone-specific (i.e., heat-labile) alkaline phosphatase, tartrate-resistant acid phosphatase, osteocalcin (BGP), procollagen peptides, and urinary hydroxyproline (1). However, many of these biochemical tests are not yet readily available to most clinicians and, more importantly, the precise role of these biochemical markers has not been firmly established. In patients with established osteoporosis (no other causes such as drugs, malignancy, or metabolic bone disease) blood BGP and urinary hydroxyproline values are often high when the osteoporosis is characterized as a "high bone turnover," form of the disease. Biochemical "testing" will be shown to have more relevance and importance in the management of the osteoporosis once a diagnosis is established.

Transiliac needle bone biopsy procedure should be reserved for those instances when more specific documentation of skeletal histodynamics is essential for diagnosis and selection of therapy. Clinical situations in which a bone biopsy may be most helpful as a diagnostic tool include instances when fractures have occurred at sites other than those commonly associated with postmenopausal osteoporosis, or when vertebral bone mass is clearly normal yet nontraumatic fractures have occurred. There is a small group of women who sustain osteoporotic fractures in the immediate postmenopausal period because of osteogenesis imperfecta or mastocytosis, diseases that often go undiagnosed without bone biopsy analysis. There are also a number of reported patients in whom a presumptive clinical diagnosis of osteomalacia has been made on the basis of the history, radiographic features, and elevated serum alkaline phosphatase, but subsequent skeletal histology has shown that the correct diagnosis was, in fact, osteoporosis. Although most of these patients report a history of gastrectomy, chronic malnutrition, inflammatory bowel disease, or drug (i.e., anticonvulsant) ingestion, it is difficult to document calcium and/or vitamin D malabsorption. Not infrequently, blood levels of 25-hydroxyvitamin D are decreased in these individuals. While bone biopsy after tetracycline administration should continue to be part of the diagnostic evaluation of this group, it should be emphasized that when the biopsy has been responsible for a change in the diagnosis, characteristically osteoporosis was diagnosed when osteomalacia was expected and not the converse.

PREVENTION

Peak adult bone mass must be optimized by ensuring an adequate dietary calcium intake during childhood and adolescence and also during the period when growth has stopped and bone accumulates at appendicular sites (11–17). Elemental calcium should be consumed at the rate of 1,500–1,800 mg/day. In reality, this is difficult for most adolescents to achieve if milk is not ingested daily, so that calcium supplements with proven bioavailability should be provided. In addition, it may be necessary to fortify the normal food chain with calcium in the same way as many foods are now fortified with vitamin D. Actually, since most teenagers are addicted to low-calcium-containing snack foods and beverages, which are usually also high in phosphate content, their eating habits should be monitored and changed accordingly (18–23). Regular load-bearing exercise will also improve bone mass during the period of bone modeling, but the optimum exercise regimen has not yet been determined (24). Once peak adult bone mass has been established, adequate calcium intake, regular exercise, and maintenance of normal estrogen/androgen function should preserve bone mass during early to mid-adult life. There is currently no known means of retarding or preventing age-related bone loss in individuals without known risk factors.

Estrogen deficiency at the menopause is the most common cause of accelerated bone loss in women and, therefore, numerically the most important pathogenetic factor in the development of osteoporosis. This is completely preventable by administration of estrogen replacement at the menopause at doses that approximate 0.625 mg conjugated estrogen for 25 days each month (1). Progesterone should also be administered along with estrogen in a cyclical regimen in dose of 5–10 mg (medoxyprogesterone) per day for 10 days per month, when the uterus is intact, in order to minimize the likelihood of estrogen-induced carcinoma of the endometrium. For those women who cannot take estrogens or who refuse to do so because of "cancerophobic" problems or because of dislike for the weight gain and/or menses that often accompany estrogen therapy, calcitonin (subcutaneous or nasal spray) can effectively replace the estrogen (25). Although calcitonin dose regimens may vary, the most effective dose regimen for the injectable form of the drug is 50–100 IU thrice weekly. Dosage requirements for nasal spray of calcitonin are usually twice those of injectable forms. Since every woman who becomes menopausal will not lose bone at an accelerated rate, it is important to assess each woman individually for her risk of developing the disease. Factors that may be helpful in this regard are listed in Table 1. The only certain means of assessing the lifetime risk of developing osteoporosis after the menopause and the need for therapy is to measure bone mass at the menopause utilizing recently developed (and commercially available) noninvasive methods of quantifying bone mass.

TREATMENT

Prevention of subsequent bone loss and prevention of falls and fractures is of paramount importance in any therapeutic menu for osteoporotic patients with established vertebral fractures. If the initial evaluation reveals a specific cause for the accelerated bone loss and vertebral fracture syndrome, this should be corrected as quickly and completely as possible. Treatment of established disease in the older patient should always be directed toward the underlying pathology. It has been well established that the skeletal histology in osteoporosis is quite heterogeneous, with the majority (about 70–75 percent) of patients demonstrating suppression of bone remodeling (so-called inactive or low-turnover osteoporosis), and the remainder demonstrating increased remodeling (active or high-turnover osteoporosis) (1). This distinction between low- and high-turnover osteoporosis has in the past been based primarily on data obtained by transiliac needle bone biopsy after *in vivo* "labeling" with oral tetracycline. One should not assume that these findings reflect a bimodal distribution of any of the histologic parameters of the dynamics of skeletal remodeling. Rather, there appears to be a continuous spectrum from low to high bone formation rates (BFR), with the majority of patients with osteoporosis having normal or low BFR. Biochemical markers of bone remodeling such as circulating BGP and urinary hydroxyproline can be used to assess the dynamics of skeletal remodeling without resorting to invasive bone biopsy procedures. The urinary hydroxyproline:creatinine ratios sampled in the second voided urine after an overnight fast of 9–12 hours are often increased in patients with high-turnover or active osteoporosis. Serum BGP is also increased in such patients, whereas blood alkaline phosphatase may prove nondiagnostic in this regard. Despite the increased specificity of some of the new assays for bone markers, there are still pitfalls in the clinical utility of each of these biochemical markers since not every patient with high turnover or active osteoporosis will show an increase in these biochemical markers, especially in the early phases.

Therapeutic agents that inhibit bone remodeling would appear to be best suited to those osteoporotic patients with vertebral fractures and high-turnover disease. Included in this category are calcium, calcitonin, and gonadal steroids (estrogen in women, testosterone in men). Although gonad steroid therapy occasionally proves effective in older women (>65–70 years of age), calcitonin appears to be the treatment of choice for this population, since, like estrogen, calcitonin initially stabilizes bone mass; in addition to this effect, calcitonin subsequently increases skeletal content. Calcitonin also has an additional advantage since it has proven analgesic potency (25). New therapeutic maneuvers such as "pulse therapy" utilizing bisphosphonates also increase bone mass and decrease fracture incidence (26). It should be emphasized that whenever one attempts to stabilize the skeleton with any drug regimen, an adequate supply of elemental calcium (i.e., 1,000–1,500 mg per day) is mandatory (27). Although vertebral bone mass appears to increase continuously for as long as 5 years in patients treated with sodium fluoride, no change in the incidence of either vertebral or hip fractures occurs, and stress fractures of the extremities often complicate the therapy. Moreover, 20–40% of patients treated with fluoride do not respond to this therapy, and the articular and/or gastrointestinal side effects mount with increasing time (28). At the time of this writing, only calcitonin and estrogen are approved by the Food and Drug Administration (FDA) for treatment of osteoporosis in the United States.

REFERENCES

1. Avioli LV, Lindsay R. Female osteoporotic syndrome(s). In: Avioli LV, Krane SM, *Metabolic bone disease and related clinical disorders*, eds. 2nd ed. Philadelphia: W.B. Saunders Co., 1990;397–451.
2. Melton LJ, Kan SH, Frye MA, Wahner HW, O'Fallon WM, Riggs BL. Epidemiology of vertebral fractures in women. *Am J Epidemiol* 1989;129:1000–1011.
3. Cummings SR, Black DM, Rubin SM. Lifetime risks of hip, Colles', or vertebral fracture and coronary heart disease among white postmenopausal women. *Arch Intern Med* 1989;149:2445–2448.
4. Mangaroo J, Glasser JH, Roht LH, Kapadia AS. Prevalence of bone demineralization in the United States. *Bone* 1985;6:135–139.
5. Prior JC, Vigna YM, Schechter MT, Burgess AE. Spinal bone loss and ovulatory disturbances. *N Engl J Med* 1990;323:1221–1227.
6. Johnston CC Jr, Hui SL, Witt RM, Appledorn R, Baker RS, Longcope C. Early menopausal changes in bone mass and sex steroids. *J Clin Endocrinol Metab* 1985;61:905–911.
7. Brody JA, Farmer ME, White LR. Absence of menopausal effect on hip fracture occurrence in white females. *Am J Public Health* 1984;74:1397–1398.
8. Phillips S, Fox N, Jacobs J, Wright WE. The direct medical costs of osteoporosis for American women aged 45 and older. *Bone* 1988;9:271–279.
9. Gilsanz V, Varterasian M, Senac MO, Cann CE. Quantitative spinal mineral analysis in children. *Ann Radiol* 1986;29:380–382.
10. Kelly PJ, Twomey L, Sambrook PN, Eisman J. Sex differences in peak adult bone mineral density. *J Bone Min Res* 1990;5:1169–1175.

11. Kelly PJ, Eisman JA, Sambrook PN. Interaction of genetic and environmental influences on peak bone density. *Osteoporosis Int* 1990;1:56–60.
12. Seeman E, Hopper JL, Bach LA, et al. Reduced bone mass in daughters of women with osteoporosis. *N Engl J Med* 1989;320:554–558.
13. Dequeker J, Nijs J, Verstraeten A, Geusens P, Gevers G. Genetic determinants of bone mineral content at the spine and radius: a twin study. *Bone* 1987;8:207–209.
14. Kelsey JL, Hoffman S. Risk factors for hip fracture. *N Engl J Med* 1987;316:404–406.
15. Bellantoni MF, Blackman MR. Osteoporosis: diagnostic screening and its place in current care. *Geriatrics* 1988;43:63–70.
16. Nevitt MC, Cummings SR, Kidd S, Black D. Risk factors for recurrent nonsyncopal falls: a prospective study. *JAMA* 1989;261:2663–2668.
17. Shah BG, Belonje B. Calcium and bone health of women. *Nutr Res* 1988;8:431–442.
18. Calvo MS, Kumar R, Heath H. Persistently elevated parathyroid hormone secretion and action in young women after four weeks of ingesting high phosphorus, low calcium diets. *J Clin Endocrinol Metab* 1990;70:1334–1340.
19. Massey LK, Wise KJ. The effect of dietary caffeine on urinary excretion of calcium, magnesium, sodium and potassium in healthy young females. *Nutr Res* 1984;4:43–50.
20. Wyshak G, Frisch RE, Albright TE, Albright NL, Schiff I, Witschi J. Nonalcoholic carbonated beverage consumption and bone fractures among women former college athletes. *J Orthop Res* 1989;7:91–99.
21. Sandler RB, Slemenda CW, LaPorte RE, et al. Postmenopausal bone density and milk consumption in childhood and adolescence. *Am J Clin Nutr* 1985;42:270–274.
22. Mann P. Teen-agers and the calcium crisis. *The Saturday Evening Post* 1987, April:68–71.
23. Calvo MS, Kumar R, Heath H III. Elevated secretion and action of serum parathyroid hormone in young adults consuming high phosphorus, low calcium diets assembled from common foods. *J Clin Endocrinol Metab* 1988;66:823–829.
24. Drinkwater BL, Bruemner B, Chesnut CH. Menstrual history as a determinant of current bone density in young athletes. *JAMA* 1990;263:545–548.
25. Avioli LV. Calcitonin therapy in osteoporotic syndromes. *JAMWA* 1990;45:103–107.
26. Storm T, Thamsborg G, Steiniche T, Genant HK, Sorensen OH. Effect of intermittent cyclical etidronate therapy on bone mass and fracture rate in women with postmenopausal osteoporosis. *N Engl J Med* 1990;322:1265–1271.
27. Heaney RP, Recker RR, Stegman MR, Moy AJ. Calcium absorption in women: relationships to calcium intake, estrogen status, and age. *J Bone Min Res* 1989;4:469–475.
28. Riggs BL, Hodgson SF, O'Fallon WM, et al. Effect of fluoride treatment on the fracture rate in postmenopausal women with osteoporosis. *N Engl J Med* 1990;322:802–809.

Calcium Nutriture for Mothers and Children, edited by
Reginald C. Tsang and Francis Mimouni. Carnation
Nutrition Education Series, Vol. 3. Carnation Co.,
Glendale/Raven Press, Ltd., New York © 1992.

Calcium Needs and Lactose Intolerance

Jay A. Perman

*Department of Pediatrics, Division of Gastroenterology and Nutrition, John Hopkins
University School of Medicine, Baltimore, Maryland 21205*

Milk is a principal source of calcium in the diet of infants, and lactose is the principal carbohydrate of milk (1). Since intolerance to lactose is common, individuals who must therefore limit their intake of milk and dairy products are likely to decrease their calcium intake concomitantly. An enhancing role of lactose in promoting calcium absorption has also been postulated, raising the possibility that restriction or absence of lactose in the diet may further impair calcium homeostasis. The controversial interrelationship of dietary calcium and lactose is examined in this discussion.

DISORDERS OF LACTOSE ABSORPTION

The physiology of lactose digestion and absorption is shown in Fig. 1, which illustrates intraluminal and intestinal mucosal processes in the digestion and absorption of dietary carbohydrates (2). Alterations of lactose digestion and absorption may be determined genetically, or result from a variety of conditions. Examples are listed in Table 1, and include ontogenetic, primary, and secondary lactase deficiency. Transient lactose malabsorption occurs in premature infants until lactase activity matures. Primary lactase nonpersistence, also known as primary lactase deficiency or primary adult-type hypolactasia, is the most clinically significant of the genetically determined causes of sugar malabsorption. This deficiency results from a postweaning decline in intestinal lactase activity. The decline begins at varying ages depending on the ethnic group but usually after age 5. The majority of the world's adult population is lactase deficient, as indicated in Table 2 (3). Paradoxically, therefore, lactase "deficiency" is the normal condition (3). Malabsorption of lactose is common in a number of intestinal diseases that cause intestinal mucosal damage or atrophy, as indicated in Table 1. These secondary causes of lactose malabsorption occur because lactase activity is the rate-limiting step in digestion of lactose (Fig. 1). Accordingly, injury to the small intestinal mucosa typically will result in lactose malabsorption while assimilation of other sugars may remain intact.

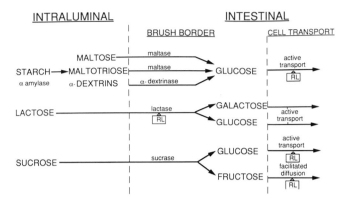

FIG. 1. Schematic diagram of absorption of dietary carbohydrate at the intestinal brush border. *RL*, the rate-limiting step in the overall digestion and absorption of the sugar. (Modified from Gray, ref. 2, with permission.)

CONSEQUENCES OF LACTOSE MALABSORPTION

Lactose malabsorption may lead to intolerance, manifested as some combination of watery diarrhea, bloating, pain, and flatulence following ingestion of the sugar. The pathophysiology of lactose malabsorption is illustrated in Fig. 2 (1). Unabsorbed lactose in the small bowel and colon exerts significant osmotic pressure, leading in some cases to a watery fecal output. A portion of the sugar entering the colon is fermented by colonic bacteria with production of lactic and other short-chain organic acids. The colonic mucosa absorbs a portion of the volatile fatty acids produced by fermentation, thereby reducing the osmotic load and thus the potential fluid loss in the stool. The extent to which these fatty acids are metabolized following their absorption also represents a salvage pathway for calories that otherwise would be lost. In addition, fermentation results in the production of the gases hydrogen, carbon dioxide, and methane, which may lead to abdominal distention and flatulence. These

TABLE 1. *Examples of lactase deficiency*

Ontogenetic
    Lactase deficiency of the premature infant
Primary
    Congenital lactase deficiency
    Primary lactase nonpersistence ("adult-onset")
Secondary
    Cow milk- and soy protein-sensitive enteropathy
    Gluten-sensitive enteropathy
    Contaminated small bowel syndrome
    Giardia lamblia infestation
    Rotavirus infection
    Short gut syndrome

TABLE 2. *Prevalence of lactose malabsorption in selected ethnic groups*

Nationality	Percent	Nationality	Percent
Americans		Danes	3
Caucasians	19	British	6
Blacks	65	Germans	15
Indians	95	Spaniards	15
Eskimos	83	Soviets (Leningrad)	15
Mexican-Americans	52	Israelis	66
Mexicans	83	Arabs	80
Canadians		Central Africans (Bantu)	95
Caucasians	6	Indians (overseas)	75
Indians	63	Vietnamese (USA)	100
Swedes	1	Thais	98

gases readily diffuse into the portal circulation and are excreted. The presence of hydrogen in expired air is an indicator of lactose malabsorption, and is discussed below.

A number of variables in addition to the digestive and absorptive capacity of an individual for lactose determines whether malabsorption produces symptoms in the given patient. These variables include residual lactase activity; the amount of lactose ingested; gastric emptying; small bowel transit; and the metabolic activity of the

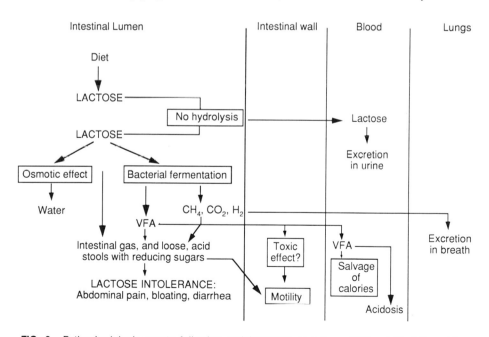

FIG. 2. Pathophysiologic events following malabsorption of lactose. *VFA*, volatile fatty acids. (From Saavedra and Perman, ref. 1, with permission.)

colonic flora toward malabsorbed lactose (1). These variables form the basis by which many individuals with lactose malabsorption attributable to "adult-onset" lactase deficiency tolerate significant amounts of milk without developing symptoms.

RELATIONSHIP OF CALCIUM NEEDS TO LACTOSE INTOLERANCE AND DIETARY RESTRICTION

Calcium nutriture may be impacted by lactose intolerance either by dietary restriction of calcium accompanying elimination of dairy products, or by the effect of lactose malabsorption on calcium absorption. It has been estimated that milk and dairy products provide 55–75 percent of the American dietary calcium supply. One quart of milk supplies approximately 1,200 mg of calcium, the RDA for a teenager. Thus, avoidance of milk and dairy products as a means of escaping the symptoms of lactose intolerance can have significant implications for calcium intake. Numerous strategies exist for modifying the symptoms of lactose intolerance without severely curtailing consumption of dairy products. Unnecessary dietary restrictions should not be advised in the absence of objective confirmation of lactose intolerance (see below).

The effects of lactose on calcium absorption remain controversial. Reasons for conflicting conclusions in investigations of the lactose/calcium relationship include inter- and intrastudy subject differences that may affect the results. For example, racial-ethnic background and age of subjects will influence brush border lactase activity. This in turn will affect luminal lactose concentrations and the luminal concentration of its hydrolytic products across individuals. The dietary intake of calcium by subjects prior to balance studies varies among investigations, and is generally uncontrolled. Moreover, methods for measuring absorption vary; some studies use traditional balance methods while others utilize radioisotopically labeled calcium.

Studies in experimental animals have suggested that the presence of lactose enhances calcium absorption (4–6). Studies in humans indicate that the apparent enhancing effect of lactose on calcium absorption may not be a function of lactose *per se* but of its hydrolytic products, glucose and galactose. Birlouez-Aragon (7) conducted a multilumen intubation study to assess the absorption of calcium in young adults given milk alone and lactase-supplemented milk. Lactose disappearance over a 20-cm length of intestine was used as an index of lactase activity. Subjects were classified either as lactase deficient or lactase sufficient according to whether there was at least a 20 percent reduction in lactose concentration at the lower collecting site compared with the upper collecting site. A linear relationship was demonstrated between the percentage of calcium absorbed and of lactose disappearance between the duodenum and jejunum during milk perfusion (Fig. 3), supporting previous data in humans indicating that the effect of lactose on calcium absorption is dependent on intestinal lactase activity (8). Lactase-deficient subjects absorbed significantly less calcium than lactase-sufficient subjects when perfused with regular milk (Fig. 4). Perfusion with lactase-supplemented milk containing the monosaccharides glu-

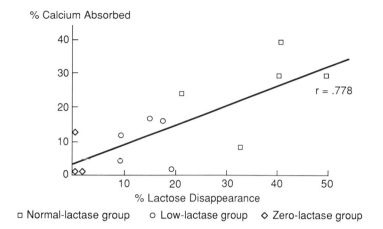

% Calcium Absorbed

% Lactose Disappearance

r = .778

□ Normal-lactase group   ○ Low-lactase group   ◇ Zero-lactase group

FIG. 3. Relationship of percent calcium absorbed versus percent lactose hydrolyzed in human volunteers with varying levels of lactase activity, utilizing perfusion of milk over a 20-cm length of upper intestine. (Modified from Birlouez-Aragon, ref. 7, with permission.)

cose and galactose significantly enhanced calcium absorption in lactase-deficient subjects, but had no effect on calcium absorption in lactase-sufficient subjects. In summary, absorption of milk calcium was significantly greater in subjects with normal lactase activity than in lactase-deficient subjects, a finding reported by others (9). Perfusion with lactase-supplemented milk enhanced calcium absorption in lactase-deficient individuals.

From these data it has been suggested that the origin of increased calcium absorption is not the lactose itself but its hydrolytic products, glucose and galactose. Birlouez-Aragon (7) interprets his results on the basis of a hypothesis by Norman et al. (10) proposing that glucose enhances calcium absorption as a consequence of water movement across the mucosa stimulated by glucose transport. The resulting concentration of unabsorbed calcium is thought to result in higher active and/or

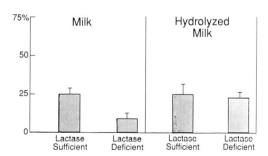

FIG. 4. Effect on calcium absorption in lactase-sufficient and -deficient individuals of hydrolysis of lactose in milk to its component monosaccharides, glucose and galactose. (Modified from Birlouez-Aragon, ref. 7, with permission.)

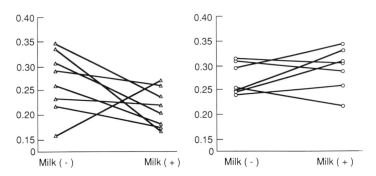

FIG. 5. Total fractional calcium absorption from milk containing lactose (+) or free of lactose and containing glucose (−). Test subjects were classified as lactase normal (**left**) or lactase deficient (**right**) on the basis of breath H_2 measurements. Data are summarized in Table 3. (Modified from Griessen et al., with permission.)

passive calcium absorption (10). Accordingly, lactose prehydrolysis could increase the absorption of calcium in lactase-deficient subjects.

However, a study by Tremaine et al. (11) comparing calcium absorption from lactose-hydrolyzed milk and unhydrolyzed milk in both lactase-deficient and lactase-sufficient individuals indicated that, within groups, there was no beneficial effect of hydrolyzed milk on absorption of calcium. In the lactase-deficient groups, calcium absorption was 33.5 percent from hydrolyzed milk and 36.2 percent from the same volume of unhydrolyzed milk. In the lactase-sufficient group, mean absorptions were 24.2 percent from hydrolyzed and 25.7 percent from unhydrolyzed milk. These differences within groups are not significant. While the data indicate that mean calcium absorption from both milks was significantly greater ($p < 0.01$) in lactase-deficient compared with lactase-sufficient individuals, presumably reflecting lower antecedent dietary calcium intake in the former, hydrolysis of lactose in the milk did not seem to have a beneficial effect on calcium absorption.

Griessen et al. (12) have confirmed the work of Tremaine et al., indicating that lactase-deficient subjects absorb calcium from standard milk better than subjects with normal lactase activity (Fig. 5). Furthermore, Griessen et al. (12) showed that these subjects absorbed calcium from lactose-free milk containing glucose as efficiently as from standard milk (Fig. 5 and Table 3). These findings are similar to those reported by Kocian et al. (13) in 1973, who reported that calcium balance did not differ when administered with standard milk or lactose-free milk containing glucose. This finding would suggest that monosaccharide resulting from lactose hydrolysis rather than lactose *per se* may be important in promoting calcium absorption, as demonstrated by Birlouez-Aragon. It would then follow that hydrolyzed products are particularly beneficial in *alactasic* individuals, in whom it could be expected that luminal glucose would be available only from exogenous hydrolysis of lactose.

Studies in infants fed lactose-free formulas have identified some differences in bone accretion and phosphorus metabolism but have largely confirmed the efficiency of calcium absorption in the absence of lactose. The effect of feeding lactose-free

TABLE 3. *Total fractional Ca absorption (TFCaA)*

	Normal lactase subjects (n = 8)			Lactase-deficient subjects (n = 7)		
	Milk with no lactose (−)	Milk with lactose (+)	p (−/+)	Milk with no lactose (−)	Milk with lactose (+)	p (−/+)
TFCaA (fraction of dose administered)	0.268 ± 0.062	0.214 ± 0.037	NS	0.270 ± 0.033	0.289 ± 0.042	NS
p (NL/LD)*					<0.01	

* Significance between normal lactase (NL) and lactase-deficient (LD) subjects for milk containing lactose.
Modified from Tremaine et al., ref. 11, with permission.

formulas on calcium homeostasis has been assessed in very low birth weight (VLBW) infants as well as term infants. In each case, the use of such soy-based formulas over time did not appear to impact calcium balance and serum levels of calcium. Shenai et al. (14) studied infants weighing 1,530 g or less in the first month of life. Calcium balance was studied utilizing 96-hour balance periods in infants fed a 24 cal/oz. soy-based formula in which the carbohydrate was a 1:1 blend of sucrose and corn syrup. Infants receiving this formula were compared with those fed a conventional 24 cal/oz milk-based formula, i.e., containing lactose. Results are shown in Table 4. Calcium absorption as a percentage of intake was comparable in the two groups as was calcium retention in mg/kg/day. In addition, serum calcium was not different between the two groups. Significant differences were, however, found in serum phosphorus, reflecting decreased phosphorus absorption in the gut in the soy-

TABLE 4. *Ca, P, N metabolism—soy versus milk[a]*

Nutrient	Intake (mg/kg/day)	Excretion (% of intake)		Absorption (%)	Retention (mg/kg/day)
		Urine	Fecal		
Calcium					
SF	136 ± 0.5	1.1 ± 0.2	54 ± 5.3	46 ± 5.3	6.1 ± 7.4
MF	129 ± 0.5	1.9 ± 0.4	47 ± 4.8	52 ± 4.8	65 ± 6.1
p	<.001	NS	NS	NS	NS
Phosphorus					
SF	78 ± 0.3	16 ± 1.9	22 ± 3.2	78 ± 3.2	49 ± 3.4
MF	96 ± 0.4	37 ± 4.1	10 ± 3.0	90 ± 3.0	51 ± 6.0
p	<.001	<.001	<.05	<.05	NS
Nitrogen					
SF	582 ± 2.2	26 ± 1.6	12 ± 1.2	88 ± 1.2	363 ± 8.9
MF	557 ± 2.0	17 ± 1.2	10 ± 0.6	90 ± 0.6	407 ± 7.4
p	<.05	<.05	NS	NS	<.05

[a] Values are means ± SEM. Absorption = intake − fecal loss. Retention = intake − (fecal + urinary loss). SF, soy-based formula group, n = 10; MF, milk-based formula group, n = 9; NS, not significant.
Modified from Kocian et al., ref. 13.

TABLE 5. *Mean serum calcium[a]*

| Age | Human milk | Formula[b] | |
		A	B
2 wk	9.9 ± 1.2	9.8 ± 1.5	9.9 ± 1.4
	(2.47 ± 0.30)	(2.44 ± 0.37)	(2.47 ± 0.35)
2 mo	10.6 ± 1.2	10.4 ± 0.8	10.9 ± 1.1
	(2.64 ± 0.30)	(2.59 ± 0.20)	(2.72 ± 0.35)
4 mo	10.5 ± 0.8	10.5 ± 1.5	10.1 ± 1.1
	(2.62 ± 0.20)	(2.62 ± 0.37)	(2.52 ± 0.27)

[a] Data arc mg/dl (mmol/l), mean ± SEM.
[b] A contains glucose polymers; B contains glucose polymers/sucrose.
Modified from Shenai et al., ref. 14, with permission.

based formula group. The authors express concern that the long-term use of soy-based lactose-free formulas, while not appearing to affect calcium homeostasis, may predispose rapidly growing neonates to phosphorus deficiency rickets.

Similarly, soy formulas free of lactose but containing glucose or glucose polymers did not affect calcium metabolism in term infants. In a longitudinal study carried out for a period of 4 months following birth, Chan et al. (15) compared soy-based formulas containing glucose polymers alone and the identical formula containing a mixture of glucose polymers and sucrose. Breast-fed infants served as lactose-ingesting controls for the two soy-formula groups. Once again, there was no difference in serum calcium expressed as mg/dl for the human milk-fed infants and the two soy formula-fed groups at 2 weeks, 2 months, and 4 months of age (Table 5). There were also no differences in serum phosphorus, magnesium, 25-OH cholecalciferol, or alkaline phosphatase values. As in the study of VLBW infants, growth was comparable over the 4 months among the various groups. In addition, bone mineral content was assessed using a bone mineral analyzer. While the soy formula-fed groups had lower bone mineral contents for the initial 4 months of the study, long-term follow-up of these infants indicated bone mineralization later became comparable to a breast-fed group. However, no comparison to a cow milk formula-fed group was made. (Table 6).

TABLE 6. *Mean bone mineral content after 6 months of age[a]*

| Age (mo) | Human milk | Formula[b] | |
		A	B
6	0.11 ± 0.02	0.08 ± 0.03	0.08 ± 0.03
12	0.14 ± 0.03	0.12 ± 0.03	0.14 ± 0.03

[a] Bone mineral content, g/cm, mean ± SEM.
[b] A contains glucose polymers; B contains glucose polymers/sucrose.
Modified from Shenai et al., ref. 14, with permission.

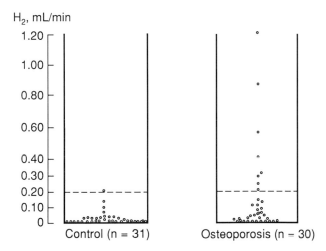

FIG. 6. Breath H_2 excretion 2 hours following lactose load in patients classified as normal or osteoporotic on the basis of bone mineral density, trabecular index, and presence of compression fractures of the vertebrae. Breath H_2 excretion greater than 0.20 ml/min was considered indicative of lactase deficiency. (Modified from Newcomer et al., ref 17, with permission.)

In contrast to these studies, which failed to demonstrate a role of lactose in promotion of intestinal absorption of calcium, Ziegler and Fomon (16) utilized balance studies to demonstrate that net absorption of calcium was significantly greater from a formula containing lactose than from one containing corn syrup solids and sucrose. Apart from differences in study design and methodology, the subjects were studied later in infancy compared with subjects in the studies noted above. Thus, the role of lactose in promoting calcium absorption from infant formulas remains controversial.

Is the *presence* of lactose detrimental to calcium absorption in lactase-deficient individuals? Among postmenopausal individuals with osteoporosis, there is a greater likelihood of lactase deficiency than in nonosteoporotic women (Fig. 6) (17), appearing to lend support to the notion that lactose could be detrimental to calcium absorption. From the evidence, it has been suggested instead that *avoidance* of dairy products containing calcium by individuals who are lactase deficient predisposes to osteoporosis. A study of lactose and calcium absorption in postmenopausal osteoporosis by Horowitz et al. (18) showed that malabsorption of lactose, detected by breath H_2 measurement, was present in 25 of 46 subjects (54 percent) studied, and not surprisingly, 76 percent of malabsorbers had gastrointestinal symptoms following lactose as compared with 14 percent of the normal absorbers (Table 7). Dietary milk intake was significantly lower in the malabsorbers than in normal absorbers. Importantly, there were no significant differences between the absorbers and the malabsorbers with respect to radioactive calcium absorption. Using the criteria of the study, malabsorption of calcium was documented in 44 percent of the lactose malabsorbers and 52 percent of the lactose absorbers. This difference is not significant.

TABLE 7. *Postmenopausal osteoporotic subjects with normal and abnormal absorption of lactose*[a]

	Lactose malabsorbers	Lactose absorbers	p
No.	25	21	—
Age (years)	65 ± 1	66 ± 2	NS
History of milk intolerance [no. (%)]	5 (20)	3 (14)	NS
Milk intake (l/wk)	1.6 ± 0.2	3.2 ± 0.7	<.025
Gastrointestinal symptoms after lactose [no. (%)]	19 (76)	3 (14)	<.01
Radioactive calcium absorption (fraction/hour)	0.65 ± 0.07	0.55 ± 0.05	NS
Malabsorption of calcium [no. (%)]	11 (44)	11 (52)	NS

[a] Data are mean ± SEM. NS, not significant.
Modified from Newcomer et al., ref. 17.

Thus, this study confirms the suspicion that osteoporosis is more likely linked with deficient intake of calcium than with calcium malabsorption. The malabsorbers tended to avoid calcium as dairy products to a greater degree than the absorbers.

DIAGNOSIS AND MANAGEMENT OF THE LACTOSE-INTOLERANT CHILD

The breath hydrogen test for lactose malabsorption forms an objective basis for modifying the child's diet in an attempt to ameliorate symptoms (19). Hydrogen (H_2) is produced in the colon and released in expired air when lactose escapes digestion in the small bowel (Fig. 2). The breath test is simple, accurate, and noninvasive, and can be performed in venues outside of the tertiary care center (3). Documentation of lactose malabsorption becomes the basis for one or more management strategies. These include: (1) reduction of lactose intake (total restriction is rarely necessary); (2) intake of lactose-reduced dairy products; (3) consumption of microbially derived lactase with lactose-containing foods; and (4) intake of autodigesting sources of lactose, e.g., yogurt. Calcium in yogurt has been shown to be well absorbed by lactase-deficient individuals, and this product is better tolerated in these individuals compared with milk containing an equal quantity of lactose (20). These approaches should conserve calcium intake without resorting to medicinal calcium supplementation.

REFERENCES

1. Saavedra JM, Perman JA. Current concepts in lactose malabsorption and intolerance. *Annu Rev Nutr* 1989;9:475–502.
2. Gray GM. Intestinal disaccharidase deficiencies and glucose-galactose malabsorption. In: Stanbury JB, Wyngaarden JB, Fredrickson DS, ed. *The metabolic basis of inherited disease,* 3rd ed. New York: McGraw-Hill, 1972;1453–1463.

3. Montes RG, Perman JA. Disorders of carbohydrate absorption in clinical practice. *MD Med J* 1990;39:383–388.
4. Ambrecht JH, Wasserman RH. Enhancement of Ca^{2+} uptake by lactose in the rat small intestine. *J Nutr* 1976;106:1265–1271.
5. Ghishan FK, Stroop S, Meneely R. The effect of lactose on the intestinal absorption of calcium and zinc in the rat during maturation. *Pediatr Res* 1982;16:566–568.
6. Miller SC, Miller MA, Omura TH. Dietary lactose improves endochondral growth and bone development and mineralization in rats fed a vitamin D-deficient diet. *J Nutr* 1988;118:72–77.
7. Birlouez-Aragon I. Effect of lactose hydrolysis on calcium absorption during duodenal milk perfusion. *Reprod Nutr Dev* 1988;28:1465–1472.
8. Cochet B, Jung A, Griessen M, Bartholdi P, Schaller P, Donath A. Effects of lactose on intestinal calcium absorption in normal and lactase-deficient subjects. *Gastroenterology* 1983;84:935–940.
9. Debongnie JC, Newcomer MD, McGill DB, Phillips SF. Absorption of nutrients in lactase deficiency. *Digest Dis Sci* 1979;24:225–231.
10. Norman D, Morawski S, Fortran J. Influence of glucose, fructose, and water movement on calcium absorption in the jejunum. *Gastroenterology* 1980;78:22–25.
11. Tremaine WJ, Newcomer AD, Riggs BL, McGill DB. Calcium absorption in milk in lactase-deficient and lactase-sufficient adults. *Dig Dis Sci* 1986;31:376–378.
12. Griessen M, Cochet B, Infante F, et al. Calcium absorption from milk in lactase-deficient subjects. *Am J Clin Nutr* 1989;49:377–384.
13. Kocian J, Skala I, Bakos K. Calcium absorption from milk and lactose-free milk in healthy subjects and patients with lactose intolerance. *Digestion* 1973;9:317–324.
14. Shenai JP, Banoo M, Jhaveri MD, Reynolds JW, Hutson RK, Babson SG. Nutritional balance studies in very low-birth-weight infants: role of soy formula. *Pediatrics* 1981;67:631–637.
15. Chan GM, Leeper L, Book LS. Effects of soy formulas on mineral metabolism in term infants. *Am J Dis Child* 1987;141:527–530.
16. Ziegler EE, Fomon SJ. Lactose enhances mineral absorption in infancy. *J Pediatr Gastroenterol Nutr* 1983;2:288–294.
17. Newcomer AD, Hodgson SF, McGill DB, Thomas PJ. Lactase deficiency: prevalence in osteoporosis. *Ann Intern Med* 1978;89:218–220.
18. Horowitz M, Wishart J, Mundy L, Nordin BE. Lactose and calcium absorption in postmenopausal osteoporosis. *Arch Intern Med* 1987;147:534–536.
19. Perman JA. Breath analysis. In: Walker WA, ed. *Pediatric gastroenterological disease*. Toronto: BC Decker Inc., 1990;1354–1362.
20. Smith TM, Kolars JC, Savaiano DA, Levitt MD. Absorption of calcium from milk and yogurt. *Am J Clin Nutr* 1985;42:1197–1200.

Calcium Nutriture for Mothers and Children, edited by
Reginald C. Tsang and Francis Mimouni. Carnation
Nutrition Education Series, Vol. 3. Carnation Co.,
Glendale/Raven Press, Ltd., New York © 1992.

Calcium and Vitamin D Requirements During Lactation: Are They Increased?

Bonny L. Specker and *Heidi J. Kalkwarf

*Department of Pediatrics, University of Cincinnati Medical Center,
Cincinnati, Ohio 45267-0541; and *Department of Neonatology, Children's Hospital
Medical Center, Cincinnati, Ohio 45299–2899*

CALCIUM

Lactation places a stress on calcium homeostasis, as approximately 200 mg/day of calcium are excreted in human milk. Due to this additional demand for calcium, dietary requirements of this mineral are thought to be higher in lactating compared with nonlactating women. The current Recommended Dietary Allowance (RDA) for calcium for adult women younger than 25 years is 1,200 mg/day, and for women older than 25 years it is 800 mg/day. The RDA for lactating women, regardless of age, is 1,200 mg/day (1).

The dietary requirement for calcium has traditionally been established using information from classical balance studies. Biochemical and outcome measurements have also been used to reflect biochemical and functional sufficiency. For example, serum concentration of 1,25-dihydroxyvitamin D [$1,25(OH)_2D$], the active vitamin D metabolite, is often used as a biochemical indicator of calcium status; concentrations of $1,25(OH)_2D$ are high during periods when calcium intake is low relative to needs. Bone mineral content or density is often used as an outcome measurement, with low bone mineral content suggesting calcium or mineral insufficiency. It has been suggested that the peak bone mass, which is attained between 20 to 40 years of age, is predictive for future development of bone fractures (2,3). As illustrated schematically in Fig. 1, the lower the peak bone mineral content or bone mass, the earlier the fracture threshold will be reached.

The questions as to whether calcium and vitamin D requirements are increased during lactation remain controversial due to discrepancies in human studies. These discrepancies may be a result of differences in study design or differences in maternal diet. The majority of studies on hormonal and bone mineral changes in human lactation have investigated women only during lactation and have used non-postpartum women as controls. However, lactation is only one part of a continuum that includes pregnancy and the postweaning period. Significant changes in calcium metabolism are known to occur during pregnancy (4), and there is recent evidence that changes postweaning also occur (5). In addition, different hormonal and bone mineral re-

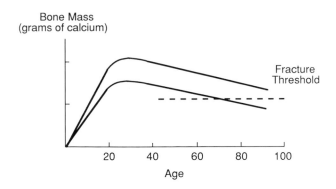

FIG. 1. Bone mass increases over the first two decades, reaching a peak during the third decade of life, and then declining. The peak bone mass attained during this period is thought to be related to the age at which a "fracture threshold" will be reached.

sponses may be expected if different amounts of calcium and vitamin D are consumed.

To help answer the question of whether there are increased calcium and vitamin D requirements during human lactation, the physiological adaptations that occur in response to the increased demand for calcium are reviewed, and evidence that reflects maternal compromises in bone mineral content during lactation is examined. In addition, evidence that addresses whether maternal dietary calcium and vitamin D influence milk concentrations of these nutrients or, consequently, the infant's nutritional status, also is examined.

Hormonal Adaptations in the Regulation of Calcium Metabolism during Lactation

The lactating mother theoretically may adapt to increased calcium loss in milk through increased intestinal absorption, decreased renal calcium excretion, and increased mobilization of calcium from bone. Under normal circumstances, the active metabolite of vitamin D, $1,25(OH)_2D$, increases the efficiency of intestinal absorption of calcium, appears to cause renal retention of calcium, and, in concert with parathyroid hormone (PTH), mobilizes calcium from bone (see the Chapter by Cruz and Tsang). Hence, elevations of $1,25(OH)_2D$ concentrations are thought to be the primary calcium-related adaptive response during lactation (6).

At the end of pregnancy, serum concentrations of $1,25(OH)_2D$ are increased, and there is a concomitant increase in calcium absorption (7). Although increases in $1,25(OH)_2D$ concentrations are seen in the lactating rat, changes in serum $1,25(OH)_2D$ concentrations observed during human lactation are not consistent. In a longitudinal study of 18 women, Greer and colleagues from Cincinnati (8) found only slight increases in serum $1,25(OH)_2D$ concentrations after 6 months of lactation. In this study, serum PTH concentrations actually decreased during lactation, and

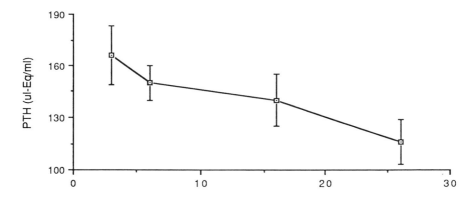

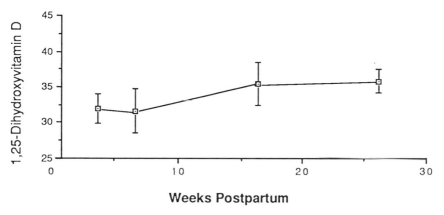

FIG. 2. Slight increases in serum 1,25-dihydroxyvitamin D [*1,25(OH)₂D*] concentrations were observed after 6 months of lactation. However, in this study serum parathyroid hormone (*PTH*) concentrations actually decreased during lactation. Thus, PTH was presumably not the stimulus to increased serum 1,25(OH)₂D concentrations. (Data from ref. 8, with permission.)

thus, PTH was presumably not the stimulus to increased serum 1,25(OH)₂D concentrations (Fig. 2). In another study, no differences in serum 1,25(OH)₂D at 6 weeks postpartum were observed in 28 lactating women when compared with 20 nonlactating postpartum women (9). These discrepancies may be a result of the controls that were used, the timing postpartum of the blood collection, and not considering dietary intake as a modifier of the hormonal responses to lactation.

There is little agreement regarding changes in PTH during pregnancy. Some studies have found that PTH increases during pregnancy (10), while others have not (11). Human data on serum PTH concentrations during lactation also are conflicting. Although PTH concentrations are elevated during lactation in rats, most studies in lactating women have found either no effect of lactation (9,12) or only a slight increase (13). If PTH concentrations increase during pregnancy, it is not clear how long they remain high postpartum regardless of lactational status. Failure to use postpartum controls may result in spurious findings, as changes observed during lactation may reflect, in part, the normal adaptive changes that occur postpartum.

Changes in calcium homeostasis during the postweaning period may play an important role in compensating for alterations in calcium balance that occur during lactation. Kent and colleagues (5) found that although PTH concentrations did not increase during lactation, they were increased at 2 months postweaning and remained elevated at 6 months postweaning. Consistent with these changes was an increased renal calcium retention postweaning.

There are only a few studies that have investigated the effect of dietary calcium on hormonal responses to lactation. Specker and coworkers (13) found significantly higher serum concentrations of 1,25(OH)$_2$D among vegetarian lactating women compared with nonlactating vegetarian women and omnivorous lactating women (Fig. 3). Mean calcium intakes among lactating vegetarian and lactating omnivorous mothers were 486 mg/day and 1,038 mg/day, respectively. It was speculated that the low calcium intake among vegetarian women resulted in an adaptive hormonal response to maximize calcium absorption. The higher serum 1,25(OH)$_2$D concentrations should theoretically increase the efficiency of intestinal calcium absorption.

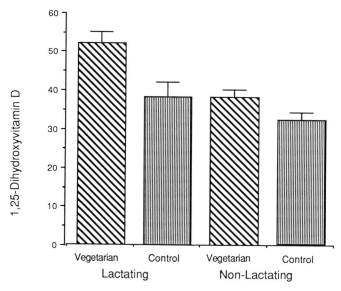

FIG. 3. Serum 1,25-dihydroxyvitamin D [*1,25-(OH)$_2$D*] concentrations in lactating vegetarian women were significantly higher than concentrations among nonlactating vegetarian women and lactating omnivorous women. (Data from ref. 13.)

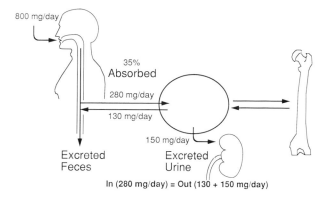

FIG. 4. The current RDA for calcium for women over 25 years of age is based on a mean intestinal absorption of approximately 35%, a mean urine excretion of 150 mg/day, and an endogenous secretion of 130 mg/day into the intestine. At an intake of 800 mg/day this would theoretically result in a "balance" between the amount going in to the body pool (280 mg/day) and the amount leaving the body pool (150 + 130 mg/day).

Calcium Absorption

The RDA for calcium is based on a mean calcium intestinal absorption of approximately 35 percent, a mean urine excretion of 150 mg/day, and an endogenous secretion of 130 mg/day of calcium into the intestine (1) (Fig. 4). Average calcium absorption in healthy nonlactating women is thought to be approximately 35 percent. Assuming that absorption does not change during lactation, lactating women would need to consume an additional 571 mg/day of calcium in order to absorb the 200 mg/day they are excreting in milk. Furthermore, this calculation also assumes that urinary calcium excretion and endogenous intestinal secretion are not affected by lactational status.

There are conflicting data as to whether calcium absorption is increased during human lactation. A 4-day calcium balance study from the 1930s observed a high net calcium absorption, similar to that observed during the last trimester of pregnancy (14). However, more recent kinetic studies, which have utilized dual tracers of calcium, have not found absorption to be increased (13,15). Classical balance studies must assume a constant endogenous secretion of calcium. The discrepancy between classical balance and dual tracer studies can theoretically be explained by changes in endogenous secretion; absorption in a classical balance study would appear to be increased if endogenous secretion decreased during lactation.

Renal Calcium Retention

Although renal reabsorption of calcium has not previously been thought to play a major role in calcium homeostasis during human lactation, recent evidence indi-

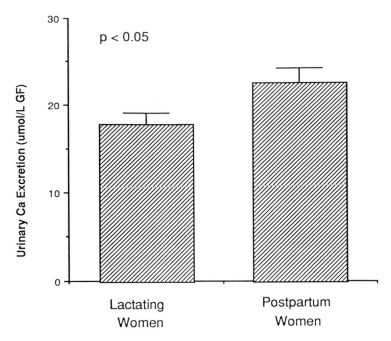

FIG. 5. A significantly lower fasting urinary calcium excretion has been observed in 40 lactating women compared with 40 non-postpartum control women. *GF,* glomerular filtration. (Data ref. 5.)

cates that it may be a major site of calcium conservation (5,6). Kent and coworkers observed a significantly lower fasting urinary calcium excretion in 40 lactating women compared with 40 non-postpartum control women (5) (Fig. 5). This renal calcium conservation was sustained throughout 6 months postweaning. These authors speculated that the increased renal reabsorption of calcium played an important role in the subsequent increase in bone mineral content postweaning. The mechanism for the renal conservation of calcium during lactation and postweaning is not clear.

Bone Mineral Content

If lactation results in a stress on the calcium status of an individual, reservoirs of calcium should theoretically be affected if insufficient dietary calcium is provided. Since 99 percent of the calcium in the body is stored in bone, it would be expected that bone should be demineralized if dietary calcium intake is low, and if the adaptive mechanisms are insufficient to compensate for the calcium demand imposed by lactation. The effect of lactation on bone mineral content has been addressed in several ways.

Cross-sectional studies have examined the bone mineral content of mothers with different histories of lactation. Some have found that bone mineral content is lower in women who breast-fed children for long periods, compared with women who did not breast-feed or breast-fed fewer numbers of children for shorter periods (16,17), while others have not found this difference (18,19). It is expected that the effect of lactation on bone mineral density should be influenced by dietary calcium intake. If dietary calcium is sufficient to meet the demands of lactation, then bone mineral should be preserved. Conversely, if dietary calcium intake is low then more pronounced effects of lactation on bone mineral density should be apparent.

Few cross-sectional studies that have examined the effect of lactation on bone mineral content have provided adequate information to assess calcium intake. Only one study in which calcium intake was reported to exceed the RDA for lactating women (1,200 mg/day) has found lower levels of bone mineral in the ultradistal forearm (primarily trabecular bone) in women who breast-fed for more than 6 months compared with women who breast-fed for less than 6 months (17). No change in cortical bone mineral of the forearm was found. In a follow-up study by the same investigators, there were no differences in bone mineral density at the lumbar, ultradistal radius, and three hip sites among women who were nulliparous (n = 10) or who breast-fed one to two children (n = 10), or who breast-fed three to four children (n = 8) (19). However, due to the large variability between subjects, the sample size may not have been large enough to pick up meaningful differences.

Walker and coworkers (18) found that multiple pregnancies and long lactations in both Bantu and Caucasian mothers were not accompanied by radiological evidence of bone loss, despite low calcium intakes. Various indices of bone density were determined from the radiographs and compared among Bantu and Caucasian mothers with large families (seven or more children) and small families (none to two children). The average daily calcium intake among Bantu mothers was 341 mg/day, while among Caucasian mothers it was 609 mg/day. There were no differences in any of the indices of bone density between mothers with large and small families or between Bantu and Caucasian mothers. However, it is possible that the radiographic methods for assessing bone loss may not be sensitive enough to detect subtle differences.

Prospective clinical studies provide more detailed information about the changes in bone density during lactation. Again, changes in bone mineral content have been reported in some studies (5,20), but not in others (21), and dietary calcium intake usually exceeded recommended levels of 800 to 1,200 mg/day. In spite of high levels of calcium intake (approximately 1,800 mg/day) a 6.5 percent decrease in trabecular bone density, but not cortical bone density, has been observed at 6 months postpartum in lactating women (20) (Fig. 6).

Kent and coworkers found that the decrease in bone mineral content that occurred during lactation was accompanied by a comparable increase in bone mineral content after weaning (5) (Fig. 7). This subsequent increase in bone mineral content appears to compensate for the loss in bone mineral that occurs during lactation. If compensation is complete, then the calcium drain invoked by lactation should not result in a net loss in bone mineral. The timing and extent to which this compensation occurs have not been well studied, but they have possible implications if pregnancies are closely spaced.

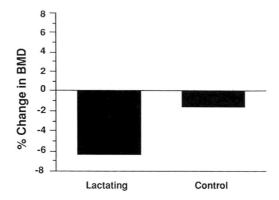

FIG. 6. In spite of high levels of calcium intake (approximately 1,800 mg/day), a 6.5 percent decrease in mean trabecular bone density (*BMD*) was observed at 6 months postpartum in lactating women. (Data from ref. 20.)

Changes in bone mineral density that may occur during pregnancy and the postweaning period may, again, explain differences between retrospective and prospective studies. An initial loss of bone mineral content early in pregnancy appears to be followed by an increase in bone mineral content later in pregnancy (7,22). Hypothetical changes in bone mineral content throughout pregnancy, lactation, and postweaning are given in Fig. 8. Thus, failure to use the appropriate postpartum control group may have led to spurious findings.

Despite adaptations that may occur in calcium metabolism and changes that occur during pregnancy and postweaning, lactating adolescent women may have an in-

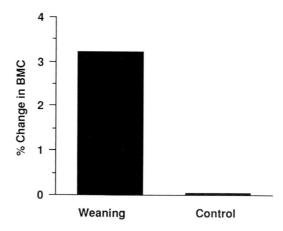

FIG. 7. Kent and coworkers found that bone mineral content (*BMC*) increased after weaning. (Data from ref. 5.)

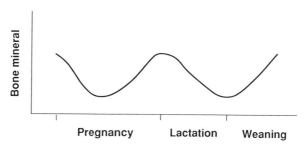

FIG. 8. Hypothetical model of changes in bone mineral content throughout pregnancy, lactation, and postweaning indicates that failure to use an appropriate postpartum control group may lead to spurious findings.

creased requirement for calcium. Calcium requirements are high for the adolescent mother due to her own growth. The additional calcium demands that pregnancy and milk production put on the mother may need to be met by increased calcium intake. A prospective intervention study in adolescent women found that the group receiving their usual intake of 900 mg calcium/day had a 10% decrease in bone mineral density at the distal forearm (primarily cortical bone) by 16 weeks postpartum, whereas there was no significant change in bone mineral density among lactating adolescent women who received at least 1,600 mg calcium/day (23) (Fig. 9).

With the exception of adolescents, there is little evidence to suggest that lactation poses a sufficient stress on calcium homeostasis such that supplemental dietary calcium is needed to preserve bone mineral content. However, conclusions regarding the effects of lactation on calcium requirements should be made with caution as there is insufficient information on changes in bone mineral content during lactation in mothers who are consuming different levels of calcium.

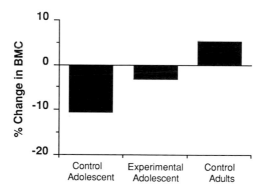

FIG. 9. Lactating adolescent women receiving their usual intake of 900 mg calcium/day (control group) had a 10 percent decrease in bone mineral content (*BMC*) at the distal forearm by 16 weeks postpartum, compared to no significant change in bone mineral density among lactating adolescent women who received at least 1,600 mg calcium/day (experimental group). (Data from ref. 23.)

Effect of Maternal Calcium Intake on Milk Concentrations

There is no evidence in adult women that a low calcium intake results in low milk calcium concentrations. Moser and coworkers found that despite 50% lower dietary intakes of calcium in Nepalese lactating women (average of 482 mg/day) compared with American lactating women, milk calcium concentrations were similar (24). Specker and coworkers (25) also observed similar milk calcium concentrations among strict vegetarian women compared with omnivorous women (27 vs. 28 mg/dl, respectively), despite different calcium intakes (486 mg/day vs. 1,038 mg/day) (25). A lower milk calcium concentration has been observed among lactating adolescents compared with lactating adult women, although the difference may be explained, at least in part, by differences in the timing of milk collections (26).

VITAMIN D

Vitamin D is synthesized endogenously in skin upon exposure to ultraviolet radiation (wavelength 280–310 nm). Utilization of the cutaneous photoendocrine system in the supply of vitamin to the body is presumably the "natural" method for acquisition of vitamin D.

Calcium balance studies conducted in the 1930s in lactating women consistently observed negative net calcium balance unless the mother's diets were supplemented with vitamin D (see ref. 6). However, during that period, routine vitamin D supplementation was not prevalent, and the negative calcium balance observed without the administration of vitamin D could have resulted from vitamin D deficiency. Whether the requirement for vitamin D is greater during lactation than in nonlactation could not be determined from these studies, as nonlactating control women were not studied and varying amounts of supplemental vitamin D were not used.

Human milk vitamin D concentrations have been found to be related to maternal vitamin D intake (27,28). Milk vitamin D concentrations are also lower in black women compared with white women (27). However, in Cincinnati, infant serum 25-hydroxyvitamin D concentrations, an indicator of vitamin D status, have not been found to be associated with either the milk vitamin D or 25-hydroxyvitamin D concentrations (27). In addition, serum 25-hydroxyvitamin D concentrations in breast-fed infants have not been found to be higher with maternal supplementation with high doses of vitamin D (29–31). It appears that in the exclusively breast-fed infant vitamin D status is more dependent upon the infant's sunshine exposure than the vitamin D content of the milk (32).

There currently are no studies indicating that supplemental vitamin D beyond the current RDA is necessary for maternal regulation of calcium during lactation or for maintaining adequate vitamin D status in the infant. The RDA of 400 IU vitamin D/day, assuming no sunshine exposure, appears to be appropriate.

ACKNOWLEDGMENTS

This work was supported in part by the Perinatal Research Institute, Cincinnati, Ohio.

REFERENCES

1. Subcommittee on the Tenth Edition of the Recommended Dietary Allowances. Food and Nutrition Board. Washington DC: National Academy Press, 1989;174–183.
2. Johnston CC, Hui SC, Wiske P, et al. Bone mass at maturity and subsequent rates of loss as determinants of osteoporosis. In: DeLuca, Frost, Webster, et al., eds. *Osteoporosis: Recent advances in pathogenesis and treatment.* Baltimore: University Park Press, 1981.
3. Matkovic V, Kostial K, Simonovic I, Buzina R, Brodarec A, Christopher Nordin BE. Bone status and fracture rates in two regions of Yugoslavia. *Am J Clin Nutr.* 1979;32:540–549.
4. Pitkin RM. Calcium metabolism in pregnancy and the perinatal period: a review. *Am J Obstet Gynecol* 1985;151:99–109.
5. Kent GN, Price RI, Gutteridge D, et al. Human lactation: forearm trabecular bone loss, increased bone turnover, and renal conservation of calcium and inorganic phosphate with recovery of bone mass following weaning. *J Bone Min Res* 1990;5:361–369.
6. Toverud SU, Boass A. Hormonal control of calcium metabolism in lactation. *Vitamin Horm* 1979;37:303–347.
7. Heaney RP, Skillman TG. Calcium metabolism in normal pregnancy. *J Clin Endocrinol* 1971;33:661–670.
8. Greer FR, Tsang RC, Searcy JE, Levin RS, Steichen JJ. Mineral homeostasis during lactation—relationship to serum 1,25-dihydroxyvitamin D, 25-hydroxyvitamin D, parathyroid hormone, and calcitonin. *Am J Clin Nutr* 1982;36:431–437.
9. Hillman L, Sateesha S, Haussler M, Wiest W, Slatopolsky E, Haddad J. Control of mineral homeostasis during lactation: interrelationships of 25-hydroxyvitamin D, 24,25-dihydroxyvitamin D, 1,25-dihydroxyvitamin D, parathyroid hormone, calcitonin, prolactin, and estradiol. *Am J Obstet Gynecol* 1981;139:471–476.
10. Pitkin RM, Reynolds WA, Williams GA, Hargis GK. Calcium metabolism in normal pregnancy: a longitudinal study. *Am J Obstet Gynecol* 1979;133:781–790.
11. Whitehead M, Lane F, Young S, et al. Interrelationships of calcium-regulating hormones during normal pregnancy. *Br Med J* 1981;283:10–12.
12. Cushard WG Jr, Creditor MA, Canterbury JM, Reiss E. Physiologic hyperparathyroidism in pregnancy. *J Clin Endocrinol Metab* 1972;34:767–771.
13. Specker B, Yergey A, Vieira N, Heubi J, Ho M, and Tsang RC. Effect of lactation and diet on calcium metabolism: stable isotope studies. *J Am Coll Nutr* 1987;6:432 (abst).
14. Toverud KU, Toverud G. Studies on the mineral metabolism during pregnancy and lactation and its bearing on the disposition to rickets and dental caries. *Acta Paediatr* 1931;12:(Suppl 2).
15. Kent N, Price R, Wilson S, et al. Increased efficiency of intestinal absorption of calcium in human pregnancy but not in lactation: absence of a correlation with serum 1,25-dihydroxyvitamin D bioavailability. *Endocrinol Soc Aust* 1989;32:98a (abst).
16. Aloia JF, Vaswani AN, Yeh JK, Ross P, Ellis K, Cohn SH. Determinants of bone mass in postmenopausal women. *Arch Intern Med* 1983;143:1700–1704.
17. Wardlaw GM, Pike AM. The effect of lactation on peak adult shaft and ultra-distal forearm bone mass in women. *Am J Clin Nutr* 1986;44:283–286.
18. Walker ARP, Richardson B, Walker F. The influence of numerous pregnancies and lactations on bone dimensions in South African Bantu and Caucasian mothers. *Clin Sci* 1972;42:189–196.
19. Koetting CA, Wardlaw GM. Wrist, spine, and hip bone density in women with variable histories of lactation. *Am J Clin Nutr* 1988;48:1479–1481.
20. Hayslip CC, Klein TA, Wray HL, Duncan WE. The effects of lactation on bone mineral content in healthy postpartum women. *Obstet Gynecol* 1989;73:588–592.
21. Byrne J, Thomas MR, Chan GM. Calcium intake and bone density of lactating women in their late childbearing years. *J Am Diet Assoc* 1987;87:883–887.

22. Purdie DW, Aaron JE, Selby PL. Bone histology and mineral homeostasis in human pregnancy. *Br J Obstet Gynaecol* 1988;95:840–854.
23. Chan GM, McMurry M, Westover K, Englebert-Fenton K, Thomas MR. Effects of increased dietary calcium intake upon the calcium and bone mineral status of lactating adolescent and adult women. *Am J Clin Nutr* 1987;46:319–323.
24. Moser PB, Reynolds RD, Acharya S, Howard MP, Andon MB. Calcium and magnesium dietary intakes and plasma and milk concentrations of Nepalese lactating women. *Am J Clin Nutr* 1988;47:735–739.
25. Specker BL, Tsang RC, Hollis B, Brazerol B. Effect of race on breast milk minerals and vitamin D concentrations. *J Am Coll Nutr* 1984;3:287–288 (abst).
26. Lipsman S, Dewey KG, Lonnerdal B. Breast-feeding among teenage mothers: milk composition, infant growth, and maternal dietary intake. *J Pediatr Gastroenterol Nutr* 1985;4:426–434.
27. Specker BL, Tsang RC, Hollis BW. Effect of race and diet on human milk vitamin D and 25-hydroxyvitamin D. *Am J Dis Child* 1985;139:1134–1137.
28. Ala-Houhala M, Koskinen T, Parviainen MT, Visakorpi JK. 25-Hydroxyvitamin D and vitamin D in human milk: effects of supplementation and season. *Am J Clin Nutr* 1988;48:1057–1060.
29. Markestad T, Kolmannskog S, Arntzen E, Toftegaard L, Haneberg B, Aksnes L. Serum concentrations of vitamin D metabolites in exclusively breast-fed infants at 70° north. *Acta Paediatr Scand* 1984;73:29–32.
30. Rothberg AD, Pettifor JM, Cohen DF, Sonnendecker EWW, Ross FP. Maternal-infant vitamin D relationships during breast-feeding. *J Pediatr* 1982;101:500–503.
31. Ala-Houhala M. 25-Hydroxyvitamin D levels during breast-feeding with or without maternal or infantile supplementation of vitamin D. *J Pediatr Gastroenterol Nutr* 1985;4:220–226.
32. Specker BL, Tsang RC. Vitamin D in infancy and childhood: factors determining vitamin D status. In: Barness, Bongiovanni, Morrow, Oski and Rudolph, eds. *Advances in pediatrics*. Chicago: Year Book Medical Publishers Inc., 1986;1–18.

Calcium Nutriture for Mothers and Children, edited by
Reginald C. Tsang and Francis Mimouni. Carnation
Nutrition Education Series, Vol. 3. Carnation Co.,
Glendale/Raven Press, Ltd., New York © 1992.

Meeting Calcium Needs with Parenteral and Enteral Nutrition in the Premature Infant

Winston W. K. Koo

*Departments of Pediatrics and Obstetrics and Gynecology, The University of
Tennessee, Memphis, Memphis, Tennessee 38163*

Preterm infants, particularly those with birth weight less than 1 kg, miss the period
of most rapid *in utero* accretion of calcium (Ca). The intrauterine accretion of Ca is
consistently above 100 mg/kg/day beyond 24 weeks' gestation and reaches a peak
of approximately 130 mg/kg/day between 30 and 34 weeks' gestation (1–4). The
recommendation for the Ca intake in small preterm infants is usually based on the
amount needed to replace the expected gains in Ca if the infant had remained *in
utero* until term gestation (3,4) and to minimize the risk for the development of
complications of poor bone mineralization, including rickets and fractures (5–7).

PARENTERAL REQUIREMENTS

In the immediate newborn period, almost all small preterm infants require a period
of Ca supplementation for the therapy of acute hypocalcemia (8). This is usually
followed by a period of parenteral nutrition (PN) beginning at 2–3 days after birth.
The duration of PN varies depending on the ability of the infant to tolerate enteral
feeding and the presence of other complications such as respiratory distress and
necrotizing enterocolitis.

The management of Ca intake of preterm infants requiring PN also should take
into account the phosphorus (P) requirements, since both are major mineral components of the skeleton and are important components of structure and function of
soft tissues. Ca (and P) needs of preterm infants receiving PN are now better defined,
with knowledge of the factors that affect the ability to maintain these minerals in
PN solutions (9–13) and *in vivo* data on the metabolic response (7,14,15) and mineral
retention (16,17).

Calcium and Phosphorus Solubility in Parenteral Solution

A number of Ca and P salts are soluble and may be used in PN, but none have
documented advantages over Ca gluconate and a mixture of sodium and potassium
mono- and di-basic phosphate salts. Higher molar concentrations of phosphate can

TABLE 1. *Factors influencing the delivery and urinary losses of Ca in parenteral nutrition*

1. Ca and P "solubility" in solution increases with:
Decreased absolute content of Ca and P
Decreased pH of amino acid–dextrose solution used
Adding P to parenteral nutrition solution before adding Ca
2. Urinary loss of Ca increases with:
Excessive infusion of Ca, fluid, glucose, sodium, amino acids, vitamin D
Phosphorus deficiency
Diuretic therapy

From Koo, ref. 20, with permission of Appleton & Lange, Inc.

be maintained in solution when Ca gluconate, instead of Ca chloride, is used as the Ca source. This is because the degree of dissociation of Ca gluconate decreases as concentration increases; thus the concentration of Ca available for precipitation when added as the gluconate salt is less than that available when added as the chloride salt (18,19). In preterm infants who received monobasic phosphate salt as the only source of P in PN solution, their blood pH was lower, i.e., increased risk for metabolic acidosis, and urine Ca excretion was higher as the mean P intake was increased from 1.0 mmol to 1.7 mmol (32 mg to 54 mg)/kg/day (17).

The maintenance of Ca and P salts in PN solution without precipitation also depends on the type and amount of other nutrients, particularly the pH of the amino acid solution and the sequence in which Ca and P salts are added to the amino acid–dextrose solution (Table 1) (20). With attention to details in the preparation of PN solutions, Ca and P can be delivered simultaneously in amounts similar to or greater than those retained by infants fed human milk (9–13). The currently recommended intakes of 12.5–15.0 mmol Ca (conversion for Ca: 1 mmol/l = 4 mg/dl) and 12.9–14.5 mmol P per liter (conversion for P: 1 mmol/l = 3.1 mg/dl) for infants requiring PN therapy (21) are shown to be stable in a 2 percent amino acid solution throughout the delivery system for the usual period of infusion (9–13). The amount of Ca and P delivered in PN solutions is described per liter in order to prevent Ca–P precipitation at high concentrations of Ca and P in PN solution (21,22). The latter results if there is fluid restriction, and the recommended intake is based on per kg body weight.

Phosphorus is present as organic phosphate in the phospholipid fraction of lipid emulsions. Each gram of 20 percent lipid emulsion contains about 0.07 mmol (2.7 mg) of P. Addition of cations directly into lipid emulsion may result in aggregation of fat droplets, and there are no data to document the safety and efficacy of the recommended concentrations of Ca (up to 15 mmol/l) and P (up to 14.5 mmol/L) when used as part of the total nutrient admixture, a technique whereby all PN nutrients are mixed and delivered from the same container (23,24).

Determination of Calcium and Phosphorus Requirement in Infants Receiving Parenteral Nutrition

The recommended Ca and P contents in PN solutions are based on recent reports on biochemical, hormonal, radiographic, and mineral balance data. Their use is as-

TABLE 2. *Approach to the use of high Ca and P content in parenteral nutrition solution*[a]

---

1. Increase by 10 percent increments daily starting at 70–80 percent of the maximum content
2. Adjust Ca and P content if necessary by daily monitoring serum Ca and P concentraton until 100 percent of desired content reached; thereafter measure serum Ca and P at 1- to 2-week intervals; measurement of renal reabsorption of P may be performed at same intervals

---

[a] 15 mM each of Ca and P; 60 mg Ca and 46.5 mg P/dl.
From Koo, ref. 20, with permission of Appleton & Lange, Inc.

sociated with stable biochemical and calciotropic hormone indices of mineral homeostasis. These include normal and stable serum concentrations of Ca, P, parathyroid hormone, calcitonin, 25-hydroxyvitamin D and 1,25-dihydroxyvitamin D, and renal tubular reabsorption of phosphate (7,14). Stepwise increase in the Ca and P content over the first 3 days of PN would minimize the risk of biochemical disturbance that may occur with a more rapid introduction of maximum mineral loading (Table 2).

PN-related bone disease is well described in adults and infants and is likely to have a multifactorial etiology although substrate deficiency, particularly of Ca and P, is important in the development of nutritional bone disease in infants (5,22,25). The severity of metabolic bone disease as indicated by biochemical and radiographic changes may be lessened when the Ca [0.68 mmol (27.2 mg)/kg/day] and P [0.61 mmol (18.9 mg)/kg/day] delivered in PN solutions is doubled (15).

Balance studies in clinically stable infants receiving 1.3–1.5 mmol (52–58 mg) Ca/kg/day and 1.1–1.3 mmol (34–40 mg) P/kg/day from PN have demonstrated that the mean fractional retention was 88–91 percent for Ca and 89–97 percent for P (16,17). Other factors such as Ca:P ratios and renal regulation of Ca and P are also important to achieve optimal mineral retention in infants receiving PN therapy.

Normally, infants are tolerant of a wide range of Ca:P ratios, as demonstrated by the apparent tolerance of the infusion of extremes of Ca:P ratio from 4:1 to 1:8 (22). However, ratios that minimized the disturbance to Ca and P homeostatic mechanism with highest Ca and P retention apply to solutions with Ca:P ratios of 1:1 to 1.3:1 by molar ratio or 1.3:1 to 1.7:1 by weight (7,14–17). A Ca:P ratio of <1:1 by weight should not be used because of potential risk for hyperphosphatemia, hypocalcemia, and other disturbances of Ca and P homeostasis (26–29).

The kidneys normally represent the main excretory route during PN, and urinary losses may have significant impact on mineral balances. For example, in an infant with a glomerular filtration rate (GFR) of 20 ml/min (28.8 l/day) and a serum Ca of 2.5 mmol/l (60 percent being ultrafiltrable), the daily amount of filtered Ca would be 43.2 mmol (864 mg). Thus, a small percent increase in renal loss of Ca would significantly alter Ca balance, particularly at the low range of Ca intake. Many factors, including P deficiency, excessive intakes of intravenous fluid, sodium, Ca, magnesium (Mg), vitamin D, and amino acids, can contribute to increased urine Ca loss (Table 1). Calciuria at >50 percent of Ca intake can occur with low Ca and P intake in PN. The calciuria with P deficiency may be improved by as much as 75 percent with an increase in P delivery to >1 mmol (31 mg)/kg/day. Cyclic PN with delivery of PN over shorter periods (10–18 hours/day) results in greater urine Ca loss compared with a continuous infusion of PN or with periods without PN infusion. Nonnutritional factors, including the use of furosemide and theophylline, can contribute to increased urine Ca loss and disturbed bone mineralization. The risk of nephrocalcinosis may also be increased during concomitant use of furosemide with high Ca and P intake from PN solutions (7,14,16–19,22,25–31).

There are no documented major complications associated with the currently recommended higher Ca [1.25–1.5 mmol (50–60 mg)/dl] and P [1.29–1.45 mmol (40–45 mg)/dl] intake for infants receiving PN (21). Serial abdominal ultrasound examination showed biliary sludge did not occur with greater frequency in infants receiving this higher Ca, P solution compared with those with lower mineral intake. Biliary sludge appeared to resolve upon enteral feeding (7,14). In the absence of chronic diuretic therapy, abnormal renal ultrasound findings have not been reported at this Ca and P intake (7,14). Aluminum, a potential toxin, is present in many intravenous nutrients, particularly the minerals (32). However, definitive evidence of aluminum toxicity has not been documented at the currently recommended Ca and P intakes.

In very small preterm infants, greater concentrations of Ca and P than could be easily maintained in PN solution may be needed to achieve intrauterine accretion of these minerals. The use of alternate infusion of Ca and P in order to increase the delivery of these minerals and to avoid Ca–P precipitation in PN solutions has been shown to result in lower Ca and P retention rates (42–63 percent) (26,27) compared with the Ca and P retention rates (73–97 percent) when Ca and P are infused simultaneously (16,17). In addition, hypercalcemia and hypophosphatemia may occur during high Ca infusion, while hyperphosphatemia and hypocalcemia may occur during high P infusion (26). Furthermore, infusion of P alone results in elevated urinary cyclic adenosine monophosphate (AMP), supporting the presence of increased circulating parathyroid hormone (26,28). Thus alternate infusions of Ca and P are not recommended. The best means to increase Ca and P retention further appears to be the early introduction of high Ca- and P-containing enteral feeding.

ENTERAL REQUIREMENTS

Enteral nutrition (EN) in preterm infants allows greater delivery of Ca and P than is possible by PN (3,4). Human milk content of Ca and P is insufficient to meet the goal of attaining intrauterine accretion rates (1–4,33–38). The evidence supporting inadequacy of mineral intake from human milk as well as standard infant milk formulas includes biochemical (low serum and urine P, elevated serum and urine Ca, and elevated serum alkaline phosphatase activity) (5,35–38) and hormonal (elevated serum 1,25-dihydroxyvitamin D) (6,39) disturbances, lower bone mineral content (40), and abnormal x-rays showing fractures and rickets (5). These abnormalities may be normalized upon Ca and P supplementation (5,35,36,39–41).

Calcium and Phosphorus Delivery in Milks

The availability in North America of lyophilized human milk powder as a supplement to mothers' milk is very limited. It has been used on an experimental basis (37,41). Human milk supplementation with individual or combination components (vitamin D, Ca, or P) has been reported (5,42–45). In view of the potential inadequacy of human milk content to match the intrauterine accretion of other nutrients (4,38), the use of Ca and P as the only supplementation for the human milk-fed small preterm infant is probably inappropriate. The most frequently used Ca and P supplementation for human milk-fed infants is a cow milk-based powder (46,47) or concentrated liquid formulation of cow milk-based preterm infant formula (48). The Ca:P ratio of commercially available human milk-fortifier and preterm infant formula is approximately 1.8:1 to 2:1 by weight and is similar to that in human milk (33,34).

Currently, most preterm infants are fed cow milk-based preterm infant formulas with high Ca, P content because of the low rate of sustained human milk feeding for these infants. The sources of Ca salt most frequently used in infant formulas are Ca carbonate, Ca phosphate tribasic, and Ca chloride (48,49). A loss of 30–40 percent of Ca and P from sedimentation in the milk, especially during continuous infusion over a period of 3–6 hours, has been reported. The mineral loss is less with newer formulations and with bolus delivery of the feeds (47,50,51).

Determination of Calcium and Phosphorus Requirements in Enterally Fed Infants

The data from balance studies using standard or stable isotope techniques, direct measurement of bone mineral content, and other studies on biochemical, hormonal, and radiographic changes of metabolic bone diseases have provided a reasonable basis for the recommendation of Ca (and P) intake in preterm infants.

Intestinal absorption and retention of Ca and P appear to depend to a large extent on the needs of the infant and are consistently higher in infants versus adults (3,52). In small preterm infants, the variability in Ca retention rate appears to depend on individual patient variability to a greater extent than the effect of body weight and postnatal age (53). Balance studies using standard and stable isotope techniques reported significant individual variability and generally high intestinal Ca absorption rates (47,50,53–59). However, the effect of gestational age on Ca absorption and retention in small preterm infants has not been clearly demonstrated.

In small preterm infants the absolute retention for Ca and P is greater with the use of higher mineral content cow milk-based milk formula designed specifically for preterm infants when compared with the use of human milk and standard milk formula with lower Ca and P content (3,35–37,41–50). When the preterm infant formulas are used to deliver 3.75–5.75 mmol (150–230 mg) of Ca and 2.45–4.13 mmol (76–128 mg) of P/kg/day, the Ca and P retention rates are consistently at or above the *in utero* value (Figs. 1 and 2). The mean fractional retention rates reported with the

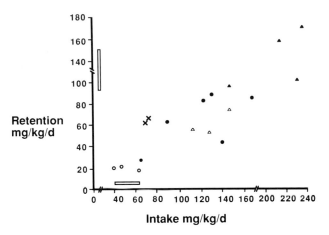

FIG. 1. Calcium retention with different nutrient sources derived from references in literature. Open circle, human milk (refs. 35, 36, 44); solid circle, human milk with various amounts of Ca and P supplement (refs. 37, 41, 44, 47, 48, 58); open triangle, low mineral-containing infant formula (refs. 36, 37, 48); solid triangle, high mineral-containing infant formula (refs. 47, 50, 58, 59); X, parenteral nutrition (refs. 16, 17); horizontal bar, range of intake from human milk at 200 ml/kg/day; vertical bar, range of *in utero* accretion. (From Koo and Tsang, ref. 31, with permission.)

use of preterm infant formulas ranged from 45 percent to 74 percent for Ca and from 54 percent to 75 percent for P (47,50,58,59). The mean fractional retention for P may be further increased to 84–92 percent in small preterm infants fed low-P milk (35,36,44).

Urinary loss of minerals also may affect mineral retention in enterally fed infants. In preterm infants fed milks with low mineral content, i.e., human milk, hypercal-

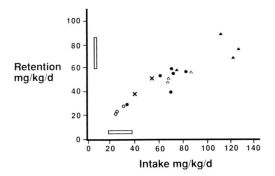

FIG. 2. Phosphorus retention with different nutrient sources derived from references in literature. Open circle, human milk (refs. 35, 36, 44); solid circle, human milk with various amounts of Ca and P supplement (refs. 37, 41, 44, 47, 48, 58); open triangle, low mineral-containing infant formula (refs. 36, 37, 48); solid triangle, high mineral-containing infant formula (refs. 47, 50, 58, 59); X, parenteral nutrition (refs. 16, 17); horizontal bar, range of intake from human milk at 200 ml/kg/day; vertical bar, range of *in utero* accretion. (From Koo and Tsang, ref. 31, with permission.)

ciuria occurs with P deficiency; P supplementation increases Ca and P retention but also increases urine P excretion. In adults, high intake of some nutrients such as protein is reported to increase urine Ca losses. However, there is no evidence that increased protein intake to the range (3.3–3.6 g/kg/day) in currently available preterm infant formulas would increase urine Ca loss. Chronic loop diuretic therapy is a major cause of increased urinary loss of minerals and increased risk of nephrocalcinosis. In contrast to their hypocalciuric effect in adults, thiazide diuretics may increase urine Ca loss in infants. Other drugs such as theophylline are also reported to increase urine Ca loss. Thus, prudence in the use of all nutrient supplements and drugs is warranted in the management of mineral intake in infants. Other nonnutritional factors such as aluminum toxicity and physical therapy may also contribute to the development of osteopenia, rickets, and fractures (22,29–32,60).

In small preterm infants within a few weeks after birth, balance studies have shown that *in utero* accretion rate can be achieved when human milk (41) and infant formulas (47,50) are fortified with Ca and P. An intake of approximately 4 mmol (200 mg) Ca and 3.2 mmol (100 mg) P/kg/day should theoretically achieve retentions of Ca and P comparable to the *in utero* accretion based on the estimated average Ca retention of 64 percent and P retention of 71 percent (3). Metabolic bone disease, as indicated by standard biochemical and radiographic findings, is reported to be less severe when preterm infants were fed mineral-fortified cow milk-based formulas with an average intake of about 5.5 mmol (220 mg) Ca and 2.8 mmol (87 mg) P/kg/day and a vitamin D supplementation of 460 IU/day for the first 7 weeks (61). These amounts of Ca and P can be provided by the two commercially available preterm infant formulas with a high mineral content.

Individual variations in mineral absorption and differences in bioavailability of mineral fortifiers may partly account for the conflicting reports on the success in matching postnatal changes in bone mineral content (BMC) to the *in utero* rate of increase in BMC as determined by photon absorptiometry (40,62,63). Studies that reported the achievement of fetal rates of increase in BMC used a total Ca intake of 210–250 mg/day and total P intake of 112–125 mg/kg/day (40,62). Thus, in selected infants, even higher amounts of mineral intake may be needed. However, complications of Ca and P containing bezoars from the Ca and P supplementation are reported (64,65). It also should be pointed out that the major problem of Ca and P deficiency with bone demineralization and rickets occurs predominantly in infants who are severely ill with multiple clinical complications (5,60). In such infants there are also practical difficulties in achieving intakes to match intrauterine mineral accretion rates.

The duration of the need for Ca and P supplementation is inversely related to the gestational age or birth weight of the infant. There are reports that a period of 6–8 weeks of increased mineral supplementation may be insufficient to prevent rickets and fractures in extremely small preterm infants with birth weights <800 g (60,66). Indeed, the occurrence of rickets and fractures is greatest at 2–4 months postnatal age and is rare after 6 months (60,67,68). Several studies have documented that by 6–9 months after birth, the BMC of small preterm infants is within the range of BMC for infants born at term, and it continues to increase throughout infancy and childhood in association with increase in skeletal size (69–71). Thus there is no physiologic rationale for Ca and P intakes to achieve the maximum *in utero* accretion rate beyond the body weights of infants born at term. For the reference preterm infant with birth weight of 1 kg, the increased Ca and P intake probably should continue for at least 3 months or until reaching a body weight of 4 kg. Thereafter, a daily intake equal to the current Recommended Daily Allowance (RDA) for term infants of approximately 60 mg/kg up to a total daily intake of approximately 800 mg at 1 year appears to be appropriate.

The use of lactose-free soy formula, in spite of its high Ca and P content, is associated with a high frequency of fractures and rickets in small preterm infants (67). Phytate in soy formula may limit P absorption (72). The beneficial effects of dietary lactose on Ca and P absorption in small preterm infants remain unconfirmed (59). Until more data are available, the use of soy formula for more than a few days in small preterm infants may be inappropriate (73).

There is no single parameter that predicts the adequacy of mineral status in small preterm infants. However, serial biochemical and radiological monitoring of skeletal development, including biweekly serum Ca, P, and alkaline phosphatase and bimonthly x-ray of forearms, can be useful for screening of rickets and fractures. Additional measurements, including serial serum concentrations of osteocalcin and calciotropic hormones and bone densitometry, may be needed to assess the adequacy of mineral status (5,19).

In conclusion, insight gained from recent studies allows a rational approach to the management of mineral intake in preterm infants receiving PN and EN. Attention to detail in the delivery of the Ca and P supplementation and in other nutritional and nonnutritional factors that affect mineral losses should maximize mineral retention and minimize the development of osteopenia, rickets, and fractures.

REFERENCES

1. Widdowson EM. Growth and composition of the fetus and newborn. In: Assali NS, ed. *Biology of gestation, vol 1, The fetus and neonate.* New York: Academic Press, 1968;1–49.
2. Ziegler EE, O'Donnell AM, Nelson SE, Fomon SJ. Body composition of the reference fetus. *Growth* 1976;40:329–341.
3. Greer FR, Tsang RC. Calcium, phosphorus, magnesium, and vitamin D requirements for the preterm infant. In: Tsang RC, ed. *Vitamin and mineral requirements in preterm infants.* New York: Marcel Dekker, 1985;99–136.
4. American Academy of Pediatrics Committee on Nutrition. Nutritional needs of low-birth-weight infants. *Pediatrics* 1985;75:976–986.
5. Koo WWK, Tsang RC. Bone mineralization in infants. *Prog Food Nutr Sci* 1984;8:229–302.
6. Koo WWK, Sherman R, Succop P, Ho M, Buckley D, Tsang RC. Serum vitamin D metabolites in very low birth weight infants with and without rickets and fractures. *J Pediatr* 1989;114:1017–1022.
7. Koo WWK, Tsang RC, Succop P, Krug-Wispe SK, Babcock D, Oestreich AE. Minimal vitamin D and high calcium and phosphorus needs of preterm infants receiving parenteral nutrition. *J Pediatr Gastroenterol Nutr* 1989;8:225–233.
8. Koo WWK, Tsang RC. Neonatal calcium and phosphorus disorders. In: Lifshitz F, ed. *Pediatric endocrinology: a clinical guide,* 2nd ed. New York: Marcel Dekker, 1990;569–611.

9. Venkataraman PS, Brissie EO Jr, Tsang RC. Stability of calcium and phosphorus in neonatal parenteral nutrition solutions. *J Pediatr Gastroenterol Nutr* 1983;2:640–643.

10. Koo WWK, Hollis BW, Horn J, Steiner P, Tsang RC, Steichen JJ. Stability of vitamin D_2, calcium, magnesium and phosphorus in parenteral nutrition solution: effect of in-line filter. *J Pediatr* 1986;108:478–480.

11. Schmidt GL, Baumgartner TG, Fischlschweiger W, Sitren HS, Thakker KM, Cerda JJ. Cost containment using cysteine HCl acidification to increase calcium/phosphate solubility in hyperalimentation solutions. *J Parenter Enteral Nutr* 1986;10:203–207.

12. Fitzgerald KA, MacKay MW. Calcium and phosphate solubility in neonatal parenteral nutrient solutions containing TrophAmine. *Am J Hosp Pharm* 1986;43:88–93.

13. Lenz GT, Mikrut BA. Calcium and phosphate solubility in neonatal parenteral nutrient solutions containing Aminosyn-PF or TrophAmine. *Am J Hosp Pharm* 1988;45:2367–2371.

14. Koo WWK, Tsang RC, Steichen JJ, et al. Parenteral nutrition for infants: effect of high versus low calcium and phosphorus content. *J Pediatr Gastroenterol Nutr* 1987;6:96–104.

15. MacMahon P, Blair ME, Treweeke P, Kovar IZ. Association of mineral composition of neonatal intravenous feeding solutions and metabolic bone disease of prematurity. *Arch Dis Child* 1989;64:489–493.

16. Pelegano JF, Rowe JC, Carey DE, et al. Simultaneous infusion of calcium and phosphorus in parenteral nutrition for premature infants: use of physiologic calcium/phosphorus ratio. *J Pediatr* 1989;114:115–119.

17. Chessex P, Pineault M, Brisson G, Delvin EE, Glorieux FH. Role of the source of phosphate salt in improving the mineral balance of parenterally fed low birth weight infants. *J Pediatr* 1990;116:765–772.

18. Lemann J Jr, Adams ND, Gray RW. Urinary calcium excretion in human beings. *N Engl J Med* 1979;301:535–541.

19. Henry RS, Jurgens RW Jr, Sturgeon R, Athanikar N, Welco A, Van Leuven M. Compatibility of calcium chloride and calcium gluconate with sodium phosphate in a mixed TPN solution. *Am J Hosp Pharm* 1980;37:673–674.

20. Koo WWK. Calcium, phosphorus and vitamin D requirements of infants receiving parenteral nutrition. *J Perinatol* 1988;8:263–268.

21. Greene HL, Hambidge KM, Schanler R, Tsang RC. Guidelines for the use of vitamins, trace elements, calcium, magnesium, and phosphorus in infants and children receiving total parenteral nutrition: report of the Subcommittee on Pediatric Parenteral Nutrient Requirements from the Committee on Clinical Practice Issues of the American Society for Clinical Nutrition. *Am J Clin Nutr* 1988;48:1324–1342.

22. Koo WWK, Tsang RC. Calcium, magnesium and phosphorus. In: Tsang RC, Nichols BL, eds. *Nutrition in infancy*. Philadelphia: Hanley and Belfus, Inc., 1988;175–189.

23. Brown R, Quercia RA, Sigman R. Total nutrient admixture: a review. *J Parenter Enteral Nutr* 1986;10:650–658.

24. Raupp P, von Kries R, Schmidt E, Pfahl HG, Gunther O. Incompatibility between fat emulsion and calcium plus heparin in parenteral nutrition of premature babies. *Lancet* 1988;1:700.

25. Koo WWK, Tsang RC. Calcium, phosphorus, magnesium and vitamin D requirements of infants receiving parenteral nutrition. In: Yu VYH, MacMahon RA, eds. *Intravenous feeding of the neonate*. London: Edward Arnold (*In press*).

26. Kimura S, Nose O, Seino Y, et al. Effects of alternate and simultaneous administrations of calcium and phosphorus on calcium metabolism in children receiving total parenteral nutrition. *J Parenter Enteral Nutr* 1986;10:513–516.

27. Hoehn GJ, Carey DE, Rowe JC, Horak E, Raye JR. Alternate day infusion of calcium and phosphate in very low birth weight infants: wasting of the infused mineral. *J Pediatr Gastroenterol Nutr* 1987;6:752–757.

28. Vileisis RA. Effect of phosphorus intake in total parenteral nutrition infusates in premature neonates. *J Pediatr* 1987;110:586–590.

29. Hufnagle KG, Khan SN, Penn D, Cacciarelli A, Williams P. Renal calcifications: a complication of long-term furosemide therapy in preterm infants. *Pediatrics* 1982;70:360–363.

30. Atkinson SA, Shah JK, McGee C, Steele BT. Mineral excretion in premature infants receiving various diuretic therapies. *J Pediatr* 1988;113:540–545.

31. Koo W, Tsang RC. Mineral requirements of low birth weight infants. *J Am Coll Nutr* 1991;10:474–486.

32. Koo WWK, Kaplan LA. Aluminum and bone disorders: with specific reference to aluminum contamination of infant nutrients. *J Am Coll Nutr* 1988;7:199–214.

33. Gross SJ, David RJ, Bauman L, Tomarelli RM. Nutritional composition of milk produced by mothers delivering preterm. *J Pediatr* 1980;96:641–644.
34. Lemons JA, Moye L, Hall D, Simmons M. Differences in the composition of preterm and term human milk during early lactation. *Pediatr Res* 1982;16:113–117.
35. Atkinson SA, Radde IC, Anderson GH. Macromineral balances in premature infants fed their own mothers' milk or formula. *J Pediatr* 1983;102:99–106.
36. Lyon AJ, McIntosh N. Calcium and phosphorus balance in extremely low birthweight infants in the first six weeks of life. *Arch Dis Child* 1984;59:1145–1150.
37. Schanler RJ, Garza C, Smith EO. Fortified mothers' milk for very low birth weight infants: results of macromineral balance studies. *J Pediatr* 1985;107:767–774.
38. Nutrition and feeding of preterm infants. Committee on Nutrition of the Preterm Infant, European Society of Pediatric Gastroenterology and Nutrition. *Acta Paediatr Scand* 1987;Suppl 336:1–14.
39. Steichen JJ, Tsang RC, Greer FR, Ho M, Hug G. Elevated serum 1,25 dihydroxyvitamin D concentration in rickets of very low birth weight infants. *J Pediatr* 1981;99:293–298.
40. Steichen JJ, Gratton TL, Tsang RC. Osteopenia of prematurity: the cause and possible treatment. *J Pediatr* 1980;96:528–534.
41. Schanler RJ, Garza C. Improved mineral balance in very low birth weight infants fed fortified human milk. *J Pediatr* 1988;112:452–456.
42. Senterre J, Salle B. Calcium and phosphorus economy of the preterm infant and its interaction with vitamin D and its metabolites. *Acta Paediatr Scand* 1982;296(Suppl):85–92.
43. Senterre J, Putet G, Salle B, Rigo J. Effects of vitamin D and phosphorus supplementation on calcium retention in preterm infants fed banked human milk. *J Pediatr* 1983;103:305–307.
44. Salle B, Senterre J, Putet G, Rigo J. Effects of calcium and phosphorus supplementation on calcium retention and fat absorption in preterm infants fed pooled human milk. *J Pediatr Gastroenterol Nutr* 1986;5:638–642.
45. Carey DE, Goetz CA, Horak E, Rowe JC. Phosphorus wasting during phosphorus supplementation of human milk feedings in preterm infants. *J Pediatr* 1985;107:790–794.
46. Greer FR, McCormick A. Improved bone mineralization and growth in premature infants fed fortified own mother's milk. *J Pediatr* 1988;112:961–969.
47. Ehrenkranz RA, Gettner PA, Nelli CM. Nutrient balance studies in premature infants fed premature formula or fortified preterm human milk. *J Pediatr Gastroenterol Nutr* 1989;8:58–67.
48. Schanler RJ, Abrams SA, Garza C. Bioavailability of calcium and phosphorus in human milk fortifiers and formula for very low birth weight infants. *J Pediatr* 1988;113:95–100.
49. Schanler RJ, Abrams SA, Garza C. Mineral balance studies in very low birth weight infants fed human milk. *J Pediatr* 1988;113:230–238.
50. Rowe JC, Goetz CA, Carey DE, Horak E. Achievement of in utero retention of calcium and phosphorus accompanied by high calcium excretion in very low birth weight infants fed a fortified formula. *J Pediatr* 1987;110:581–585.
51. Bhatia J. Formula fixed. *Pediatrics* 1985;75:800–801.
52. Food and Nutrition Board, National Research Council. *Recommended dietary allowances*. Washington, DC: National Academy Press, 1989;174–194.
53. Cooke RJ, Perrin F, Moore J, Paule C, Ruckman K. Nutrient balance studies in the preterm infant: crossover and parallel studies as methods of experimental design. *J Pediatr Gastroenterol Nutr* 1988;7:718–722.
54. Moore LJ, Machlan LA, Lim MO, Yergey AL, Hansen JW. Dynamics of calcium metabolism in infancy and childhood. I. Methodology and quantification in the infant. *Pediatr Res* 1985;19:329–334.
55. Ehrenkranz RA, Ackerman BA, Nelli CM, Janghorbani M. Absorption of calcium in premature infants as measured with a stable isotope ^{46}Ca extrinsic tag. *Pediatr Res* 1985;19:178–184.
56. Hillman LS, Tack E, Covell DG, Vieira NE, Yergey AL. Measurement of true calcium absorption in premature infants using intravenous ^{46}Ca and oral ^{44}Ca. *Pediatr Res* 1988;23:589–594.
57. Liu Y-M, Neal P, Ernst J, et al. Absorption of calcium and magnesium from fortified human milk by very low birth weight infants. *Pediatr Res* 1989;25:496–502.
58. Raschko PK, Hiller JL, Benda GI, Buist NRM, Wilcox K, Reynolds JW. Nutritional balance studies of VLBW infants fed their mothers' milk fortified with a liquid human milk fortifier. *J Pediatr Gastroenterol Nutr* 1989;9:212–218.
59. Wirth FH Jr, Numerof B, Pleban P, Neylan MJ. Effect of lactose on mineral absorption in preterm infants. *J Pediatr* 1990;117:283–287.

60. Koo WWK, Sherman R, Succop P, et al. Fractures and rickets in very low birth weight infants: conservative management and outcome. *J Pediatr Orthoped* 1989;9:326–330.
61. Laing IA, Glass EJ, Hendry GMA, et al. Rickets of prematurity: calcium and phosphorus supplementation. *J Pediatr* 1985;106:265–268.
62. Greer FR, Steichen JJ, Tsang RC. Effects of increased calcium, phosphorus, and vitamin D intake on bone mineralization in very low-birth-weight infants fed formula with Polycose and medium-chain triglycerides. *J Pediatr* 1982;100:951–955.
63. Modanlou H, Lim MO, Hansen JW et al. Growth, biochemical status, and mineral metabolism in very-low-birth-weight infants receiving fortified preterm human milk. *J Pediatr Gastroenterol Nutr* 1986;5:762–767.
64. Cleghorn GJ, Tudehope DI. Neonatal intestinal obstruction associated with oral calcium supplementation. *Aust Paediatr J* 1981;17:298–299.
65. Koletzko B, Tangermann R, von Kries R, et al. Intestinal milk-bolus obstruction in formula-fed premature infants given high doses of calcium. *J Pediatr Gastroenterol Nutr* 1988;7:548–553.
66. Cooke RJ. Rickets in a very low birth weight infant. *J Pediatr Gastroenterol Nutr* 1989;9:397–399.
67. Callenbach JC, Sheehan MB, Abramson J, Hall RT. Etiologic factors in rickets of very low birth weight infants. *J Pediatr* 1981;98:800–805.
68. Lyon AJ, McIntosh N, Wheeler K, Williams JE. Radiological rickets in extremely low birthweight infants. *Pediatr Radiol* 1987;17:56–58.
69. Helin I, Landin LA, Nilsson BE. Bone mineral content in preterm infants at age 4 to 16. *Acta Paediatr Scand* 1985;74:264–267.
70. Greer FR, McCormick A. Bone mineral content and growth in very-low-birth-weight infants. Does bronchopulmonary dysplasia make a difference? *Am J Dis Child* 1987;141:179–183.
71. Koo WWK, Sherman R, Succop P, et al. Sequential bone mineral content in small preterm infants with and without fractures and rickets. *J Bone Miner Res* 1988;3:193–197.
72. Shenai JP, Jhaveri BM, Reynolds JW, Huston RK, Babson SG. Nutritional balance studies in very low birth weight infants: role of soy formula. *Pediatrics* 1981;67:631–637.
73. Soy-protein formulas: recommendations for use in infant feeding. Committee on Nutrition, American Academy of Pediatrics. *Pediatrics* 1983;72:359–363.

Calcium Nutriture for Mothers and Children, edited by
Reginald C. Tsang and Francis Mimouni. Carnation
Nutrition Education Series, Vol. 3. Carnation Co.,
Glendale/Raven Press, Ltd., New York © 1992.

The Assessment of Bone Mineral Status and Mineral Dietary Adequacy

Russell W. Chesney

Department of Pediatrics, The University of Tennessee, Memphis; and Le Bonheur Children's Medical Center, Memphis, Tennessee 38103

During childhood, the skeleton undergoes a series of changes that ultimately result in mature adult stature. For adult stature to be achieved, a coordination of many factors must occur, including adequate intake of minerals; physiological regulation of these minerals by the kidney, intestine, and bone; appropriate concentrations of ions in the extracellular fluid; and regulation of these processes by complex hormonal control. The ultimate importance of all these processes for reaching peak bone mass during childhood and adolescence as a preventive force of osteoporosis later in life was recently recognized at a Consensus Conference at the National Institutes of Health (1).

Humans have a growth pattern similar to other primates (2). Rapid growth occurs during fetal life and then decelerates during the neonatal period and infancy. Between the second and third years of life, a steady growth rate is achieved that continues until puberty, when a characteristic growth spurt occurs. Growth ceases when the epiphyseal plates of the long bones close (3). These growth phases are indicated by a varying growth rate per annum, that is, 20–26 cm in the first year, 10 cm in the second, and 5–8 cm annually until puberty when the growth rate rises to 10 cm/year and ultimately ceases about 4–5 years after puberty (4). A critical factor in linear growth is bone growth. Moreover, the ultimate determinant of adequate mineral metabolism is the quantity of mineral in bone, termed the *bone mineral content* (BMC) (5). Because as much as 99 percent of total body calcium and 80–85 percent of phosphorus are present in the mineral phase of bone, deficiencies in the extracellular concentration of these minerals are reflected by reduced BMC and, therefore, diminished bone mineral status. This chapter reviews current methods by which bone mineral status can be measured.

Historically, bone mineral status was measured by conventional roentgenography, but this method is far too imprecise to permit a careful evaluation of BMC (5). Although the quantity and density of bone mineral can now be evaluated by many methods (6), single-beam photon absorptiometry (SPA) has been the most widely used technique since its clinical introduction in 1976 following development in the 1960s (7). Bone mineral mass and density can be determined noninvasively by other absorptiometric techniques including dual-photon absorptiometry (DPA), quantitative computed tomography (QCT), and dual-energy x-ray absorptiometry (DEXA) (8,9).

SINGLE-BEAM PHOTON ABSORPTIOMETRY

SPA measurements of the long bones have been the preferred method to assess skeletal status in infants and children (5,10) (Figs. 1 and 2). Advantages include the rather low radiation dose (<10 mrem), which is limited to the scan site, so that serial measurements can be used to study age-related changes in BMC (5); assessing the efficacy of therapy to reverse demineralization (11–13); and the correlation of long bone measurements with total body calcium as measured by the neutron activation technique (14,15) (Fig. 3).

Largely because of unreliable methods such as x-ray, the assessment of neonatal bone mineral accretion rate and the accurate diagnosis of osteopenia was difficult until the SPA technique was developed. Conventional radiological methods detect demineralization only if a 30–40 percent reduction in bone loss exists (16). Quantitative techniques, including radiological photodensitometry and radiological morphometry, require unacceptably high doses of x-irradiation for the child (17,18). Biochemical measurements of serum calcium, phosphate, magnesium, and alkaline

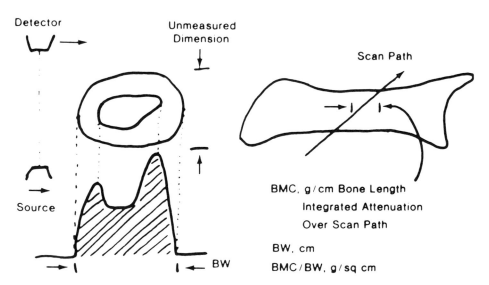

FIG. 1. Schematic diagram of radiation source and detector, demonstrating passage across midshaft of bone and the way in which bone mineral content (*BMC*) and bone width (*BW*) are determined. Although the scan path through the bone shaft appears oblique, the source and detector actually pass across the bone shaft transversely. Note that the area under the curve is directly proportional to BMC and that the attenuation of the photon beam is caused by bone mineral. (From ref. 5, with permission.)

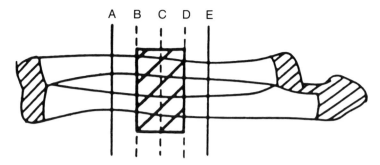

FIG. 2. Site C represents the mid-shaft. The section of stable BMC is between A and D. Beyond D (proximal direction), BMC changes significantly with distance. In practice, the measurement site falls between B and C (i.e., in the center of the section of stable bone). Hatched area designates the section of bone excised for ashing. (From ref. 10, with permission.)

phosphatase activity, as well as serum calcitriol, calcidiol, and parathyroid hormone values, do not always accurately reflect bone mineral status.

SPA data have been reported for healthy neonates of all gestational ages (15,19,20) and healthy children of 1–6 (21) and 5–20 years old (22–27). Data have also been derived for children with various conditions associated with bone disorders, including anticonvulsant therapy (28), renal disease (11,12,29), hypocalcemic and hypophosphatemic rickets (30,31), cystic fibrosis (32), diabetes mellitus (33,34), asthma (M. Brenner, personal communication), and growth hormone deficiency (35).

SPA consists of a highly collimated monoenergetic photon beam emitted from a relatively low energy (<70 keV) source that is moved at a constant speed across the bone of interest (5) (Fig. 1). Most typically, [125]I (27 keV) is used to measure forearm bones (5). Because of the small size of bones in children, a beam size at the source opening of 1–3 mm is used (8). Low energy ensures a good contrast between bone and soft tissue. This distinction is especially important in the preterm infant whose BMC may be quite low compared with term neonates and infants. The forearm is wrapped in a tissue-equivalent material to give a constant soft tissue thickness. Photon radiation transmitted through the soft tissue and bone is measured with a collimated scintillation detector. The transmitted counts are transformed by a computer, and photon beam attenuation by both bone and soft tissue are compared. An integral of the area under the absorption curve is directly proportional to mineral mass in the cross-sectional area of the scanned bone. The mineral mass, in grams, is then expressed for a 1-cm longitudinal length of long bone to derive the BMC, which is then expressed in grams per centimeter. The BMC normalized for the size of bone, or its width (BW), is expressed as bone mineral density, or the BMC/BW (grams per square centimeter) (36). We will use the term BMD to represent this ratio of BMC/BW.

Early commercial SPA devices were linear scanners that measured density along a single line with an analog computer. The scanning site was at a point one-third of the distance of the forearm, proximal to the radial epiphysis (10) (Fig. 2). Over 95

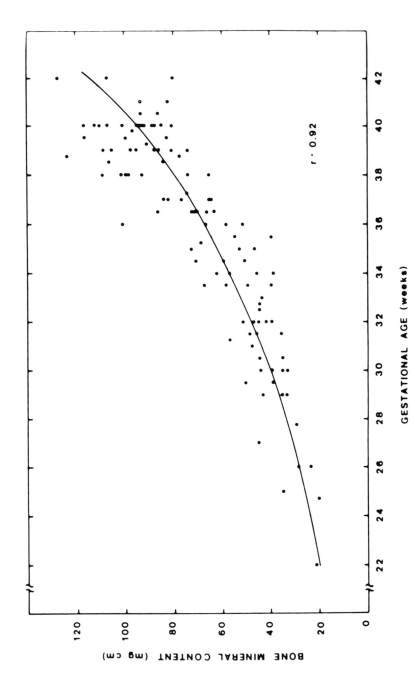

FIG. 3. Bone mineral content in the distal radius compared with gestational age. Data derived from preterm and term neonates of gestational age shown on the abscissa. (From ref. 15, with permission.)

percent of bone at this site is compact bone; 5 percent is cancellous bone (37). Error was lessened by multiple passes (usually four) over a single scanning site, which were then averaged.

The introduction of microcomputers to SPA devices permits control of scanner movement as well as analysis and normalization of digital data (38). The scanner apparatus can measure multiple contiguous scan lines in a rectilinear pattern over an area several centimeters in length. This key advance over linear scanners is important because it provides a more precise measurement that averages anatomical variation. Rectilinear scanners can also be used to determine BMC at more distal sites on the forearm and the os calcis, which contain greater proportions of trabecular (or cancellous) bone (39). Precision errors for rectilinear scanners in adults (1–2 percent for the radius at midshaft or one-third sites and 3 percent for more distal sites) are about one-half of those found with linear scanners (38).

It is necessary to modify commercial SPA devices to scan infants because of their size and poorly mineralized bone; this low BMC is even more relevant for the preterm infant (15,19). Such problems also beset the measurement of the humerus, which has twice the BMC of the radius (21). A prototype SPA unit for infants, developed at the University of Wisconsin Bone Mineral Laboratory, features a computer-based, digital readout system, high accuracy and precision, direct readout of BMC and BW, automatic data calibration, and an even lower activity source (<50 mCi ^{125}I) (15). Typical modifications needed to set up an infant device are shown in Table 1 and include scan speed changes, collimation, source activity (weaker), and step interval (15). The limit of detectability is about 0.02–0.03 g/cm after these adaptations (19). Infants can be measured easily when special tables and forearm holders are used. The radiation dose is approximately 10 mrem. The error of the method is perhaps 4 percent (15).

A midshaft site is preferable to distal one-third sites in infants because bone mineral change per millimeter is the least at this site, and repositioning errors are minimized (10) (Fig. 2). The radius is easier to measure than the humerus, particularly because slight body movements lead to large precision errors in humerus measurements.

The SPA measurement of the radius in neonates of varying gestational age permits

TABLE 1. *Modifications made in densitometry adapted for infants*

	Infant	Adult
Detector		
Collimation (mm)	1–2	3
Scan speed (mm/sec)	0.25–0.4	1.5
Step interval (mm)	0.5–1	3
Lines	4–6[a]	4[b]
Source activity (mCi)	20–50	50–200

[a] Overlaid.
[b] Contiguous.

establishment of the normal intrauterine rates of bone mineralization (15,19,21). Greer et al. (15) make the point that measuring BMC in preterm infants permits the development of "intrauterine" curves of bone mineralization in the fetus (15) (Fig. 4). Photon absorptiometry can also be used to measure bone width, thus documenting appositional bone growth (40) (Fig. 5). Greer (41) has used this technique to document that relatively poor bone mineralization, as compared with the intrauterine curve (15) (Fig. 4), occurs in very low birth weight infants after birth, regardless of their diet or the presence or absence of bronchopulmonary dysplasia (15) (Fig. 6). Mimouni and Tsang (42) discuss utilization of the intrauterine curves developed by Greer et al. (15) and Minton et al. (19), which are similar in shape. They further point out that expression of results in terms of BMC and BW permits assessment of bone mass growth versus growth of bone size being scanned. They criticize the use of the BMC/BW ratio as an unproven conceptual adjunct, which confers no specific advantage and which could mask specific information about bone mass and size (42).

Several groups have stressed the suitability of humerus scanning in infants (43,44). This site can easily be palpated (43), used to develop intrauterine curves (44), and used in longitudinal studies to evaluate the efficacy of treatment (44). Furthermore, very low birth weight infants may be more successfully scanned when the humerus is scanned because bone mineral per centimeter is approximately twice as great in the humerus as in the radius (15,43,44).

SPA has been used to compare the BMC achieved after ingesting different formulas. Chan et al. (45) studied 40 full-term, soy-based formula-fed infants in contrast to human milk-fed infants and found a reduced BMC in soy-fed infants at 2 months and 4 months, but not at 2 weeks, 6 weeks, 6 months, and 12 months. Steichen and Tsang (46) found reduced BMC in soy-based formula-fed infants compared with cow milk formula-fed infants at 6 months and 1 year but not earlier. Bainbridge et al. (47) concluded that in term infants in whom the use of soy-based formula is indicated (such as for proven lactose intolerance or cow milk allergy), soy-based formula appears to be a reasonable substitute for cow milk-based formulas, at least in terms of growth and bone mineralization (47). In other studies comparing BMC in preterm infants fed human milk, cow milk-based formula, or soy-based formula, BMC was not different at 12 months when humeral BMC was evaluated (48,49) (Fig. 7). All of these studies (45–48) and Greer's review article (41) note no real increase in BMC over the first 6–9 months of life, even though BW is increasing; therefore, the BMC/BW actually declines initially (40) (Figs. 8 and 9). At 9–12 months, there is an increase in BMC, and "bone mineral density" also increases (42).

The use of mineral supplementation for either fortification of human milk or in a "humanized" mineral-enriched formula may result in higher BMC values at 2 weeks and 3–4 weeks after initiation of diet in preterm infants whose birth weight was under 1,500 g (50). In this study BMC was measured at the distal one-third radius; significant increases in BMC were seen only in those infants fed mineral-enriched premature infant formula (50). Chan et al. (51) compared three formulas to human milk in 36 preterm infants weighing under 1,600 g. They compared distal one-third radius values in infants fed human milk and formulas containing 117.0 mg of calcium (Ca) and 58.5

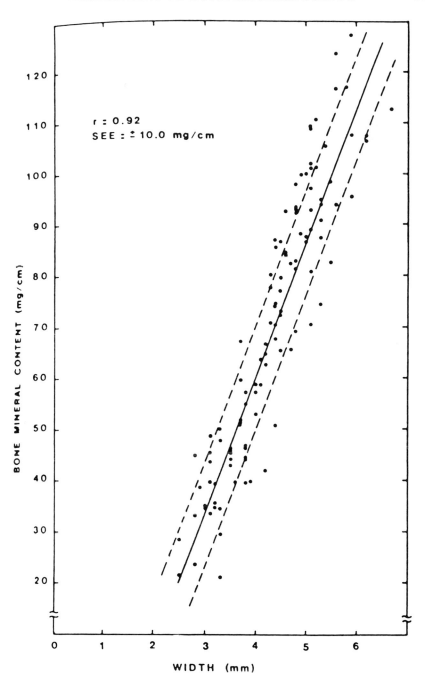

FIG. 4. Bone mineral content versus bone width as measured by photon absorptiometry in the left radius of 114 newborn infants of all gestational ages. Dotted lines represent ± SEE. (From ref. 15, with permission.)

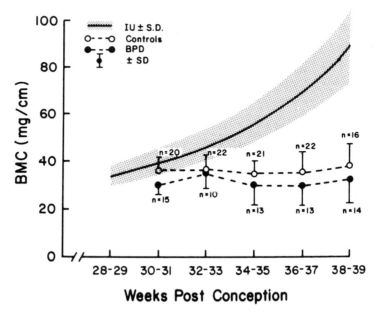

FIG. 5. Bone mineral content (*BMC*) measured in milligrams per centimeter by photon absorptiometry versus weeks postconceptional age in growing very low birth weight premature infants with bronchopulmonary dysplasia (*BPD*) and without BPD (control subjects). Unbroken, shaded line represents intrauterine (*IU*) change in BMC ± SD. (From ref. 40, with permission.)

mg of phosphorus (P) per 100 kcal; 117.0 mg of Ca and 82.0 mg of P; and 140.0 mg of Ca and 82 mg of P. BMC was higher in all formula-fed infants. All human milk-fed infants had a decline in BMC over the 2-week study despite a comparable weight gain and caloric intake (51).

Thus, since its introduction, SPA has been useful in the evaluation of BMC and bone density of term and preterm infants (51,52). However, it has also been useful in the evaluation of bone mineral status in older children. A large body of normative data in healthy children between the ages of 1 and 6 years (21) and in older children (11,22–27) is available (Fig. 10). By using radial measurements, the Wisconsin group measured BMC in more than 100 normal infants (15) (Fig. 3) and in approximately 1,000 healthy subjects between the ages of 5 and 20 years (23–25). Normal control values from Wisconsin (15,23–25) and Scandinavia (26) were largely derived from white subjects. In the study performed in Cincinnati in younger children (21), a slightly but significantly increased BMC was found in young boys compared with young girls. In the Wisconsin normative data (23–25), this gender difference was not apparent until the onset of puberty, such that at the end of adolescence, the average boy had a 35 percent increase in radial BMC compared with girls (11) (Fig. 10). Because children grow at different rates and usually have growth spurts at various times within a given year, it is necessary to use factors other than chronological age as a variable. Thus, in many studies of BMC, this measurement at each site was

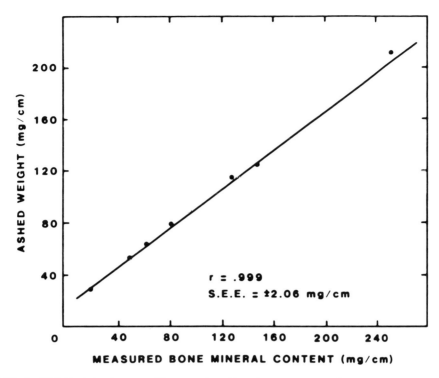

FIG. 6. Weight of nine 1-cm small bone sections (three from premature infants, six of avian origin) after ashing versus bone mineral content as measured by photon absorptiometry. (From ref. 15, with permission.)

determined for each patient in relation to an appropriate chronological age, sex, height, weight, and bone width in control subjects with a computer program that performs a multivariate analysis utilizing multiple correlation coefficients (23–25,29–33). This program can be adapted to a personal computer so that after entering the age, sex, height, weight, BMC, and BW of a child, one can determine the BMC of that child relative to an ideal subject (5). The BW and BMC determined can then be compared with an ideal subject (5), obtaining an appropriate control value to derive a normalized BW and BMC for radius, ulna, and humerus. The percent of BMC (that is, the percent of expected normal) for all three bone sites was determined by averaging this percentage at all three sites. The multiple correlation coefficient for height, weight, sex, age, and BW in relation to BMC was 0.85–0.9; the standard error of estimate is 6–10 percent, depending on the age of the subject. If the standard error of estimate is taken as being roughly equivalent to the standard deviation, then the BMC can be expressed in standard deviation scores (SD score or Z-score). Similarly, one can determine the SD or Z-score for height (53). Using this notation system, a decline of approximately 2 standard errors of estimate (-2 Z) for BMC and of -2 Z for height was considered indicative of significant osteopenia and height reduction, respectively (5).

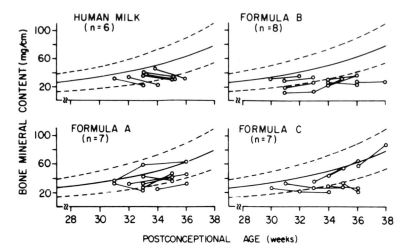

FIG. 7. Bone mineral content of four feeding groups: human milk and formulas A, B, and C. Curve represents intrauterine bone mineralization. Broken lines represent 5th and 95th tolerance limits, respectively; and solid line indicates 50th percentile. (From ref. 49, with permission.)

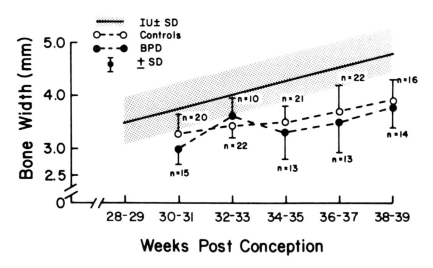

FIG. 8. Bone width measured in millimeters by photon absorptiometry versus weeks postconceptual age in growing very low birth weight premature infants with bronchopulmonary dysplasia (*BPD*) and without BPD (control subjects). Unbroken, shaded line represents intrauterine (*IU*) change in BW ± SD. (From ref. 40, with permission.)

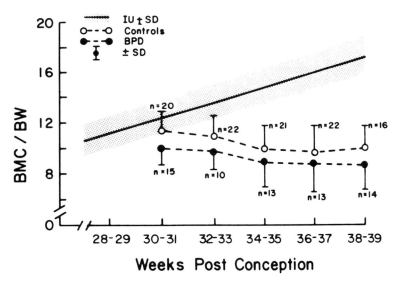

FIG. 9. Ratio of bone mineral content (*BMC*) to bone width (*BW*) versus postconceptional age, calculated from values used in Figures 5 and 8, for bronchopulmonary dysplasia (*BPD*) and control infants. Unbroken, shaded line represents intrauterine (*IU*) change in BMC/BW ratio ± SD. (From ref. 40, with permission.)

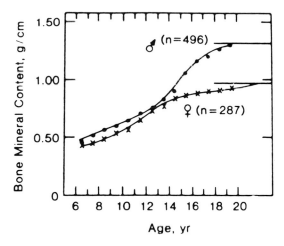

FIG. 10. Bone mineral changes of age in radial shafts of Wisconsin children. The coefficient of variation of BMC was 10 percent at each age. (From ref. 11, with permission.)

Chesney et al. (11,12) have studied the influence of renal disease on the skeleton of the growing child, particularly because the vitamin D–endocrine axis involves the kidney (54). They have used SPA to study both BMC and the BMC/BW ratio in children who have a variety of renal disorders including exposure to long-term glucocorticoid therapy for chronic glomerulonephritis (12,13), and following renal transplantation (55). In a cross-sectional study, significant demineralization, that is, -2 SD, was found in 42 percent of the 74 children evaluated (11). It is of particular interest that significant demineralization was evident in 75 percent of children with tubulointerstitial disease. Despite relatively normal renal function or only minimal impairment of glomerular filtration rate, as evidenced by a serum creatinine concentration under 1.0 mg/dl, 14 of the total 74 children in the study who took glucocorticoids were demineralized. In seven children, changing the dosage from daily to alternate-day prednisone therapy resulted in an increase in the previously reduced BMC (12,13).

The children with glomerular disorders were more critically examined (11–13,55,56). These children, who acquired renal diseases other than congenital disease, were further divided into two groups: group 1 patients, who had predominantly the steroid-responsive form of nephrotic syndrome, received short-term (up to 4 weeks) or long-term (over months to years), alternate-day prednisone at doses up to 2.7 mg/kg/48 h; and group 2 patients, including those who had active nephrotic syndrome, mesangiocapillary glomerulonephritis, or other chronic glomerular conditions, did not receive glucocorticoids. Significant demineralization was found in 18 of 25 prednisone-treated group 1 patients and none of the group 2 patients ($p < 0.001$). Group 1 subjects (-0.8 ± 0.1 SD) were shorter than control subjects, whereas group 2 patients (-0.3 ± 1.0) were not significantly shorter ($p < 0.02$). Height velocity was 2.6 ± 0.8 cm/yr in group 1 patients (0.45 height velocity SD score) versus 5.8 ± 0.8 cm/yr (0.81 height velocity SD score) in group 2 patients ($p < 0.05$). After discontinuation of prednisone therapy, six group 1 patients had an increase in BMC and height toward normal over the course of the next 6–12 months (12) (Fig. 11). This study indicates that BMC and height velocity are correlated and that both are influenced by glucocorticoid therapy rather than glomerular disease *per se,* particularly in children whose serum creatinine is less than 1.0 mg/dl.

In children with a severe reduction in renal function, radiologically demonstrable renal osteodystrophy, hypocalcemia, and a reduction in serum 1,25-dihydroxyvitamin D_3 [1,25(OH)$_2$D$_3$] concentrations, BMC was significantly diminished (53). Treatment with oral calcitriol (1,25(OH)$_2$D) resulted in an increase in forearm BMC at a rate of approximately 1 percent per month during year 1 of therapy (56,57) (Fig. 12).

To assess bone mineral status over a longer time interval, we determined BMC in 48 children with chronic renal disease over a period of 2–6 years (56). Again, patients exposed to glucocorticoids over a 15-month to 10-year period had greater demineralization and a lower rate of growth despite having a lower serum creatinine concentration than patients not taking glucocorticoids. No correlation was found between BMC and height velocity (expressed as centimeters per year) or with cal-

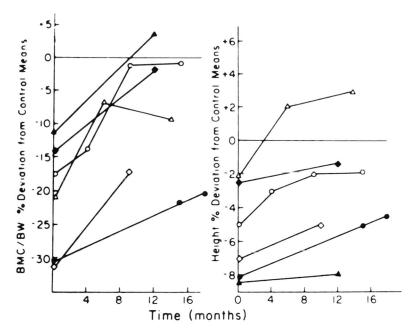

FIG. 11. Changes with time in bone mineral content/bone width (*BMC/BW*) ratio and height after prednisone therapy was discontinued. The patient designated by the solid triangle has closed epiphyses and therefore did not grow. Other patients were younger. (From ref. 12, with permission.)

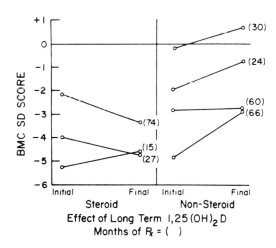

FIG. 12. The influence of oral 1,25(OH)$_2$D$_3$ on bone mineral content (*BMC*) Z-score in patients receiving or not receiving glucocorticoids. The number in parenthesis represents the number of months on therapy. (From ref. 57, with permission.)

culated creatinine clearance in either group 1 or 2. However, BMC and height Z-score correlated greatly.

Over the interval from 15 months to 10 years of follow-up in the steroid-responsive patients, many parameters tended to remain constant: initial and final height Z-score, initial and final BMC Z-score, and initial and final BMC for low (<1.2 mg/dl) or high (>1.2 mg/dl) serum creatinine values. Although therapeutic intervention with oral calcitriol improved BMC in group 2 patients by at least 0.5 Z-score (57) (Fig. 12), it did not improve the Z-score in the three group 1 patients also treated with this active vitamin D metabolite. This unexpected tendency for BMC and height Z-scores to remain constant over time for a given child on steroids is an interesting finding requiring further study.

These findings led us to examine our patients who underwent renal transplantation (55). On the one hand, they experienced a restoration of renal function, but, on the other, they had continuous exposure to glucocorticoids. BMC was evaluated in 18 children for a total of 783 months after successful transplantation. Eleven children (61 percent), aged $3\frac{7}{12}$ to $17\frac{1}{2}$ years, showed a BMC below -2 Z-score in 55 of 89 measurements (62 percent). This bone loss was progressive; among 10 of the 16 patients followed serially for more than 2 years, 5 had no change and only 1 demonstrated improvement. No correlation was found between BMC and the use of furosemide, type of transplant, prior form of renal disease, need for a repeat graft, chronic anticonvulsant treatment, or serum calcium and phosphate concentration. BMC was inversely correlated with serum creatinine concentration ($p < 0.001$) and prednisone dose (mg/kg/24 h; $p < 0.001$). Patients receiving prednisone on alternate days had a significantly higher BMC Z-score than those patients receiving prednisone daily. This prolonged and progressive bone demineralization may indicate that renal transplant patients treated with glucocorticoids are at risk for acquiring disabling bone disease. Whether the same is true in children whose antirejection therapy consists predominantly of cyclosporine A has not been established.

The studies of children with renal disease discussed suggest that glucocorticoid therapy is associated with a real reduction in BMC that is reversed only by discontinuing these steroids. Furthermore, it is helpful to see how SPA is used to assess bone mineral status in children in these studies. Appreciable changes in BMC Z-scores are readily evident from SPA assessments and thus serve a useful tool in the clinical setting.

Chesney and colleagues (28,31,32,34,58) also examined a number of pediatric patients with disorders that may induce hypomineralization or demineralization. Among those studied are diabetes mellitus (34), cystic fibrosis (32), Turner's syndrome (58), growth hormone deficiency (35), anticonvulsant osteomalacia (28), and X-linked hypophosphatemic rickets (31). Each condition was associated with a significant reduction in BMC Z-score in an appreciable number of subjects (57), with a sequential decline in BMC evident over time (5,57). Calcitriol therapy was effective in increasing BMC in ten children with X-linked hypophosphatemic rickets who were followed for at least 24 months because radial spine BMC rose by 0.9 ± 0.2 SD (31). The main conclusion to be drawn from these studies is that bone mineral status can be assessed in a cross-sectional fashion in a variety of conditions and that SPA can be used to assess the effect of therapy in a longitudinal fashion. Further studies can address the effect of "tight control" insulin therapy in BMC in patients with diabetes mellitus or the effect of estrogen administration on BMC in patients with Turner's syndrome over time.

Other pediatric conditions that demonstrate demineralization have been assessed by SPA. Reduced bone mineral content, which is responsive to testosterone therapy, has been reported in adolescent hypogonadism (59). Anorexia nervosa can also influence skeletal mineral composition, although the loss in spine mineral detected by DPA is greater than bone loss in the forearm detected by SPA (60). The short-term use of oral phosphate and calcitriol $(1,25(OH)_2D_3)$ with regard to BMC was evaluated in a group of subjects with X-linked hypophosphatemia (61). This study was noteworthy because investigators compared SPA with combined cortical thickness (CCT) of the second metacarpal and QCT of vertebral trabecular bones. In these subjects with X-linked hypophosphatemia, mineralization defects, although undetected by QCT, were detected by SPA and CCT. Short-term treatment with phosphate and calcitriol did not improve BMC.

DUAL-PHOTON ABSORPTIOMETRY

DPA has proved to be an accurate and precise method for evaluating bone mineral in the axial and total skeleton (62–65); however, the lengthy scan time required (20–60 minutes versus 2 minutes with SPA) increases the likelihood of movement errors with this method. DPA has not been widely used in children, and the data base in normal children is limited (66). Additionally, DPA's relatively larger beam size has increased the difficulty in measuring small bones.

An advantage of DPA is the potential for reassessing body composition (fat, lean body mass). DPA has been used in children at risk for anticonvulsant osteomalacia (67) and with renal disease (68,69); children with renal osteodystrophy had nearly identical bone loss when forearm SPA measurements were compared with DPA measurements of total body bone and spine mineral. Children receiving glucocorticoid therapy for glomerulonephritis had greater spine mineral loss (68,69). Finally, some investigators feel that DPA may be effectively used in investigating metabolic bone disease and endocrine disorders in children (66). This viewpoint is based on the theoretical consideration that many of these conditions are associated with demineralization.

Other conditions in pediatric patients studied by DPA include anorexia nervosa (70) and normal control subjects (71). DPA was particularly useful in anorexic subjects because it could not only measure spine and femur BMC but also assess fat content and lean body mass. An absolute decrease in total body BMC was evident in anorexic subjects compared with young, healthy women. The total body BMD was also reduced, indicating that density was low even after accounting for the reduced skeletal size (70). DeSchepper et al. (71) described a linear increase in BMD

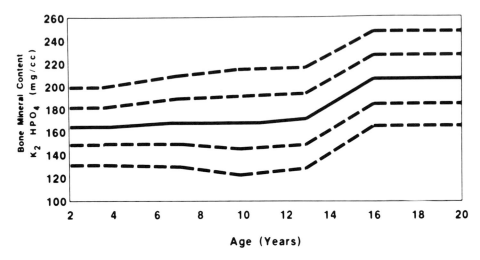

FIG. 13. Percentiles for trabecular vertebral density in children 2 to 20 years of age. (From ref. 72, with permission.)

in lumbar spine in a small number of healthy children as the children aged (71) (Fig. 13). Pubertal status was not recorded.

QUANTITATIVE COMPUTED TOMOGRAPHY

QCT has also been used to measure BMC in children (72). This technique has the potential to ascertain important information about the relative degree of mineralization of cortical and trabecular bone in infants and children. However, the extraction of quantitative information from a QCT image of the spine requires intricate calibration, rigorous quality control, and a scanning procedure of greater complexity than either SPA or DPA. The typical precision error of QCT in adults is 4–9 percent, which is greater than the 1–3 percent with DPA or SPA. Nevertheless, QCT is unique in that it permits noninvasive measurement of the characteristics of cortical and trabecular bone simultaneously. The specific technique used is computerized tomography (CT). Each study takes approximately 10 minutes, and radiation exposure is considerable, i.e., on the order of 200 mrem, which is 50 percent of a regular CT head study (72). Because the marrow of children contains little fat compared with adults, the accuracy of QCT in measuring bone mass is actually greater in young children than in adults.

Normative data for QCT bone mineral content in the first two decades of life are available and were obtained from previously examined children who required abdominal CT studies because they suffered acute trauma (73) and vertebral bone density peaks at the cessation of linear growth and with epiphyseal closure (72) (Fig. 14). It is of interest that Gilsanz et al. (73) find that spine bone density measured as

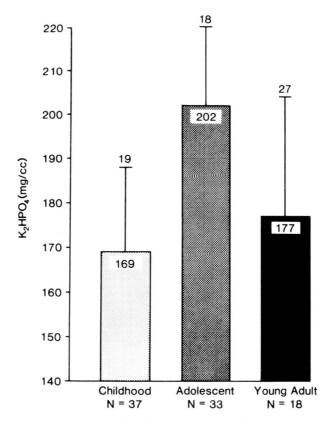

FIG. 14. Comparison between the trabccular vertebral density of Caucasian prepubertal children, adolescents, and young adults. Young adults have significantly less vertebral density than do adolescents. (From ref. 72, with permission.)

K_2HPO_4 (mg/cm^3) is similar in both boys and girls, whether prepubertal or pubertal (72) (Fig. 15). Thus, the differenccs in spine BMC and bone density must occur after growth has ceased. Gilsanz also finds a decline in trabecular vertebral density when comparing adolescents and young adults; he suggests that this decline in bone mass may reflect the reduction in physical activity between adolescents and adults (72).

QCT has been used to survey children with acute lymphoblastic leukemia (ALL) (74). ALL survivors had significantly reduced spine trabecular bone mineral density compared with age-, gender-, and race-matched nonleukemic control subjects. The decline in bone density as determined by QCT was not observed by a subset of subjects who had received cranial irradiation; disease *per se* or chemotherapy was not a risk factor for demineralization.

Osteopenia and reduced trabecular bone density were also found in children with cystic fibrosis (75) (Fig. 16). The decline in bone density was unrelated to age; the Shwachman clinical evaluation score appeared to predict subjects who were demin-

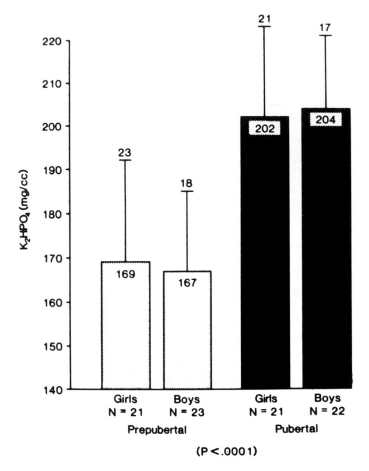

FIG. 15. Mean and standard deviations for bone density of prepubertal and pubertal children. Differences between the groups are highly significant. (From ref. 72, with permission.)

eralized, and greater disease was correlated with greater demineralization. Demineralization was also common in patients with poor nutrition. These findings are similar to those reported by Mischler et al. (32), who evaluated BMC with SPA. This technique will undoubtedly have greater application in the future.

DUAL-ENERGY X-RAY ABSORPTIOMETRY

DEXA (also called DPX) is a major new development in bone densitometry. With this method, a dual-energy x-ray source is substituted for the radionuclide source used in SPA or DPA (9,76). Because x-ray sources have a greater radiation flux, this method gives better precision (~1 percent), improved image resolution (<1 mm),

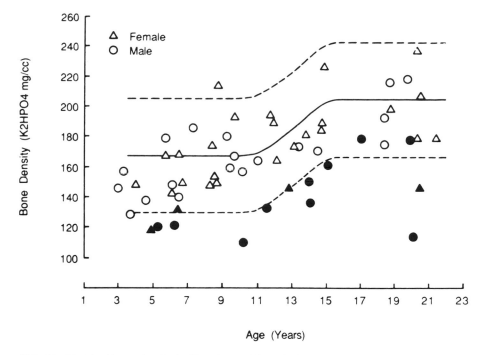

FIG. 16. Vertebral bone density in 57 patients with cystic fibrosis plotted against normal curve and 95 percent confidence interval. Darkened symbols denote presence of osteoporosis using conventional chest radiography. (From ref. 75, with permission.)

and more rapid scan times (5 to 10 times more rapid than DPA) (8). The radiation dose is as low or even lower than that used with SPA or DPA because the beam is highly collimated and optimal for bone contrast. An advantage of DEXA over single-energy, x-ray absorptiometry is that it does not require a tissue-equivalent material around the limb of the infant or child (9). Both regional bone mineral and total body calcium can be measured simultaneously by DEXA. Total bone mineral in the peripheral skeleton can also be measured. Commercial DEXA devices incorporate spine, femur, and total body algorithms found on most DPA devices. The results are comparable to DPA scans but are more precise and rapid. DEXA uses two basic techniques: (1) a stable x-ray tube with constant voltage can be used with a K-edge filter to produce a dual-energy beam, such as a cerium filter, which produces an effective 40 and 70 KeV (77); and (2) the alternate system switches rapidly between high and low KeV settings, which can produce fluctuations in output and effectiveness. However, devices using this switching technique compensate for these fluctuations on a pixel-by-pixel basis by placing a rotating wheel containing known reference materials in the beam (77).

DEXA has been used to measure BMC of the lumbar spine in 146 normal children (78). Correlations were made with age, height, weight, body surface, bone age, pubertal status, calcium intake, and vitamin D status. BMC was also correlated with serum osteocalcin values. BMC increased from 0.446 ± 0.048 g/cm^2 at year 1 to 0.891 ± 0.123 g/cm^2 at year 15, the greatest increase occurring at the time of puberty. At age 12, spine BMC was equal between boys and girls, a finding similar to those reported for radius BMC measured by SPA (5) and spine BMC measured by QCT (72). BMC by DEXA did not correlate with vitamin D or calcium intake.

Because of low radiation dose, the short time required for scanning, and the high precision of DEXA, this technique should be widely used and will be helpful in the investigation and long-term follow-up of children with diseases that impair bone metabolism.

ULTRASOUND

Attenuation of broad-band ultrasound and the speed of sound have been used to measure bone "density" in growing animals, adult humans (79), and human neonates (80). Wright et al. (80) measured sound transmission velocity (SVC) and compared their findings with midshaft forearm BMC as measured by SPA. SVC through the distal radius and ulna increases linearly with gestational age and SVC is reliably correlated with midshaft BMC. Although the precision error was only 2 percent, it corresponds to a value of 35 m/sec or about 50 percent of the speed of sound through bone. If this precision error can be reduced to under 10 m/sec, this technique may prove useful (8).

WHICH CHILD TO SCAN?

The obvious question after discussing methods of assessing bone mineral status is: which child should undergo scanning? The answer is complex and several aspects must be evaluated. First, before beginning any program of bone scanning in children, it is important to have normal values obtained from healthy children. Although many devices provide control values, the population of children on which these are based may differ appreciably from your own population. For example, differences in height, weight, race, and age at the onset of puberty may influence "normal" BMC or BMD (5).

Second, the investigator may wish to perform a cross-sectional or a longitudinal study. The latter type is obviously more important in the long-term follow-up of a single patient or a group of patients, or to assess the influence of therapy or a deleterious event in the course of a disease. Third, an investigator may wish to evaluate a normal population such as rapidly growing preterm infants, healthy newborns, or adolescent males and/or females. Hence, the population of interest will answer the question posed at the beginning of this section.

In addition, an investigator can list a number of disorders in which the assessment of BMC or BMC may be of value either in appreciating the degree of bone demin-

TABLE 2. *Disorders in childhood possibly resulting in dimineralization*

Chronic renal insufficiency
Vitamin D-dependent rickets, type I
Vitamin D-dependent rickets, type II
Familial hypophosphatemic rickets
Cystic fibrosis
Turner's syndrome
Kleinfelter's syndrome
Steroid-induced osteopenia
Asthma
Chronic glomerulonephritis
Nephrotic syndrome
Inflammatory bowel disease
Growth hormone deficiency
Leukemia
Lymphoma
Diabetes mellitus
Anorexia nervosa
Chronic active hepatitis
Drugs
Anticonvulsants
Steroids

eralization or evaluating therapeutic intervention. The conditions that should be considered are indicated in Table 2.

ASSESSMENT OF DIETARY MINERAL ADEQUACY

Current methods for assessing dietary mineral adequacy in infants and children are imprecise and are as follows: (1) the assessment of mineral intake; (2) measurement of the amount of mineral (calcium and/or phosphate) absorbed by the gastrointestinal tract; and (3) the urinary and stool excretion of minerals. Pitfalls exist in each of these areas. Because the amount of mineral retained depends on an accurate measurement of each component, the errors are compounded (8).

Assessing dietary mineral intake depends on direct measurement of the dietary consumption of foods and an accurate measurement of the calcium and phosphate in the food ingested (81). Measuring calcium and phosphate intake is relatively straightforward in the neonate and infant, particularly in those who are formula fed because the mineral content and volumes can be directly measured (82). Several factors, however, affect calcium intake in this age group. First, calcium concentrations in human milk are significantly lower than in cow milk and vary with the stage of lactation (83); longitudinal studies show a linear decline in calcium content over the duration of lactation (84).

Human milk contains calcium at 240–260 mg/l and declines to 170 mg/l by 21 months (83,84). Calcium is distributed between the lipid and aqueous fractions; indeed, up to 10 percent of total calcium is associated with the human fat globule membrane (85). The relative fat intolerance of preterm and term infants can thus theoretically affect calcium absorption. Furthermore, in gavage- or tube-fed infants, the fat globules may layer on the tubing sides, resulting in reduced intake of calories and minerals (86). While intake volume and content may be determined accurately, the volume of burped milk or vomitus is difficult to measure accurately. When compiling these data, even under ideal circumstances, the intake of calcium may be imprecisely estimated.

Phosphorus content of human milk is also lower than cow milk phosphate levels (87). Phosphorus content declines from 147 mg/l to 107 mg/l by 26 weeks (87). Bovine milk contains 930 mg of phosphorus/l, and commercial formulas provide 330–390 mg/l. The distribution of phosphorus and organic phosphates is not well described, although some are in the nucleosides and nucleotides in the diet (88). The absorption and retention of formula phosphates have been shown to be more complete than in either human or cow milk (81). Indeed, modified cow milk formulas will increase the serum phosphorus concentration to a significant degree (89). This elevation in serum phosphate concentration can also lead to an elevation of serum immunoreactive parathyroid hormone (PTH).

The absorption of both calcium and phosphorus by the neonatal or infantile intestine is quite high, particularly in terms of calcium absorption (90). Schanler et al. (82) have shown retentions of 86 percent and 80 percent for calcium and phosphorus in a group of very low birth weight infants fed a mineral-supplemented human milk formula. They reviewed a group of nine balance studies of calcium and phosphorus intake, absorption, and retention in very low birth weight infants fed human milk (82). Calcium intake varies from 40 to 92 mg/kg/day and phosphorus from 24 to 62 mg/kg/day. Calcium absorption varies from 27 to 71 mg/kg/day or 34–80 percent and phosphorus absorption from 22 to 58 mg/kg/day or 86–95 percent. Retention is 18–63 mg/kg/day or 21–53 percent and 21–53 mg/kg/day or 69–92 percent, respectively, for calcium and phosphorus. These studies indicate that the calcium retention rate does not approach the intrauterine rate of 120–150 mg/kg/day (91).

Evaluation of dietary mineral adequacy in the older child and adolescent is also problematic because of these same factors; that is, there is difficulty in assessing mineral intake, conducting balance studies, and estimating urinary losses.

It can also be difficult to measure accurately the intake of food in children. The 24-hour dietary recall, the 72-hour recall, and time-spaced food frequency measurements are typical methods used to assess nutrient intake (92). The 24-hour recall is valuable in assessing day-to-day variability in macronutrient intake. A significant correlation between the 24-hour recall and weighed food intake has also been noted (93). Fortunately, with regard to calcium intake, a strong correlation exists between dietary recall methods and a food frequency questionnaire (94). However, the recall of dietary intake by parents can be inaccurate (95). For this reason, it is better to perform consensus recall. Recently, the use of electronic methods, including recording onto a tape via the telephone, has been shown to be equivalent to parental 24-hour recalls (96). The 3-day diet recall method is probably superior to food frequency recall methods particularly regarding calcium intake (97). Specific to certain types of patient groups, food use may be underestimated (97) or overestimated by these techniques (95). Finally, if the gold standard is the precise measurement of food intake on a metabolic ward, all other methods suffer (95,97).

Estimation of phosphate intake in the child and adolescent is also problematic because these children ingest a large amount of carbonated beverages that use phosphoric acid as a component (98). Accurately assessing the intake of these beverages is difficult because children often drink portions of a can or bottle. Candies also contain large amounts of phosphate, which vary greatly in quantity (98). Children consume dairy products as a large portion of their diet, but again, because of differences in processing, the actual quantities of calcium and phosphate differ.

A complete discussion of intestinal absorption of calcium and phosphate and its evaluation is beyond the scope of this chapter. Other chapters in this text have focused on the physiology of mineral absorption. The fundamental problem in evaluating intestinal absorption of calcium in children is that the investigator cannot use radiolabeled calcium to evaluate this process directly (99,100) because of federal research regulations that protect minors. Furthermore, stable isotope studies are extremely expensive and not readily available. Thus the investigator is forced to estimate absorption using classical balance techniques (82). The errors in balance studies are many, as discussed above.

Urinary excretion of calcium and phosphate can be assessed accurately; a variety of nomograms are available to define calcium and phosphate excretion, as reviewed by Bijvoet (101). Again, a discussion of the methods for expressing urinary calcium and phosphorus excretion is beyond the scope of this chapter. However, phosphate excretion is usually defined as the percent of tubular reabsorption of phosphate (%TRP) or the tubular maximum reabsorption for phosphate [$TmPO_4 \div$ glomerular filtration rate (GFR)]. The derivation of these formulas are elegantly discussed by Bijvoet (101). Calcium excretion is usually expressed as milligrams per kilograms of body weight per 24 hours or as the calcium/creatinine ratio (102). The fundamental problem, however, is that obtaining a complete urine collection in an infant or child is very difficult. Thus, measuring daily calcium or phosphate excretion frequently underestimates the actual amount excreted.

Measuring calcium and phosphate in stools is also problematic. The stool collection is difficult unless a patient is in a metabolic unit; a relative difficulty is in finding technical staff to measure minerals in stool samples. Thus the measurement of calcium and phosphate balance is flawed and is, at best, an estimate of actual intake, absorption, and excretion.

ACKNOWLEDGMENTS

Sincere appreciation to Brenna Nichols for expert editorial assistance.

REFERENCES

1. Peck WA, Riggs BL, Bell NH, et al. Research directions in osteoporosis. *Am J Med* 1988;84:275–282.

2. Rimion DL, Horton WA. Short stature. Part 1. *J Pediatr* 1978;92:523–528.
3. Sissons HA. The growth of bone. In: Bourne DH, ed. *The biochemistry and physiology of bone,* vol 3. New York: Academic Press, 1971;143–161.
4. Royer P. Growth and development of bony tissues. In: Davis JA, Dobbing J, eds. *Scientific foundations of paediatrics.* Maryland: University Park Press, 1981;565–589.
5. Chesney RW, Shore RM. The noninvasive determination of bone mineral content by photon absorptiometry. *Am J Dis Child* 1982;136:578–580.
6. Cameron JR, Sorenson J. Measurement of bone mineral in vivo: an improved method. *Science* 1963;142:230–232.
7. Mazess RB, Cameron JR. Skeletal growth in school children: maturation and bone mass. *Am J Phys Anthropol* 1971;35:399–408.
8. Mazess RB, Barden HS, Bisek JP, Hanson J. Dual-energy x-ray absorptiometry for total body and regional bone-mineral and soft tissue composition. *Am J Clin Nutr* 1990;51:1106–1112.
9. Barden HS, Mazess RB. Bone densitometry in infants. *J Pediatr* 1988;113:172–177.
10. James JR, Truscott J, Congdon PJ, Horsman A. Measurement of bone mineral content in the human fetus by photon absorptiometry. *Early Hum Dev* 1986;13:169–181.
11. Chesney RW, Mazess RB, Rose P, Jax DK. Bone mineral status measured by direct photon absorptiometry in childhood renal disease. *Pediatrics* 1977;60:864–872.
12. Chesney RW, Mazess RB, Rose P, Jax DK. Effect of prednisone on growth and bone mineral content in childhood glomerular disease. *Am J Dis Child* 1978;132:768–772.
13. Chesney RW, Rose PG, Mazess RB. Effect of prednisone on growth and bone mineral content in childhood glomerular disease. *Pediatrics* 1984;73:459–466.
14. Cohn SH, Ellis KJ, Caselnova RC, Letteri JM. Correlation of radial bone mineral content with total body calcium in chronic renal failure. *J Lab Clin Med* 1975;86:910–919.
15. Greer FR, Lane J, Weiner S, Mazess RB. An accurate and reproducible absorptiometric technique for determining bone mineral content in newborn infants. *Pediatr Res* 1983;17:259–262.
16. Griffiths HJ, Zimmerman RL, Barty A, Snider R. The use of photon absorptiometry in the diagnosis of renal osteodystrophy. *Radiology* 1973;109:277–281.
17. Lachman E. Osteoporosis: the potentialities and limitations of its roentgenologic diagnosis. *Am J Radiol* 1955;74:712–715.
18. Mazess RB, Cameron JR, Sorenson JA. A comparison of radiological methods for determining bone mineral content. In: Whedon GD, Cameron JR, eds. *Progress in methods of bone mineral measurement,* U.S. publication no. DHEW:455–479. Washington, DC: U.S. Department of Health, Education, and Welfare, 1970.
19. Minton SD, Steichen JJ, Tsang RC. Bone mineral content in term and preterm appropriate-for-gestational-age infants. *J Pediatr* 1979;95:1037–1042.
20. Steichen JJ, Kaplan B, Edwards N, Tsang RC. Bone mineral content in full-term infants measured by direct photon absorptiometry. *AJR* 1976;126:1284–1285.
21. Vyhmeister NR, Linkhart TA, Hay S, Baylink DJ, Ghosh B. Measurement of bone mineral content in the term and preterm infant. *Am J Dis Child* 1987;141:506–510.
22. Specker B, Brazerol W, Tsang R, Levin R, Searcy J, Steichen J: Bone mineral content in children 1 to 6 years of age: detectable sex differences after 4 years of age. *Am J Dis Child* 1987;141:343–344.
23. Hui SL, Johnston CC Jr, Mazess RB. Bone mass in normal children and young adults. *Growth* 1985;49:34–43.
24. Mazess RB, Cameron JR. Growth of bone in school children: maturation and bone mass. *Am J Phys Anthropol* 1971;35:399–408.
25. Mazess RB, Cameron JR. Growth of bone in school children: comparison of radiographic morphometry and photon absorptiometry. *Growth* 1972;36:77–92.
26. Mazess RB, Cameron JR. Bone mineral content in normal U.S. whites. In: Mazess RB, ed. *Proceedings of the First International Conference on Bone Mineral Measurement,* DHEW publication no. 74-683. Washington, DC: U.S. Department of Health, Education, and Welfare, 1974:228–238.
27. Landin L, Nilsson BE. Forearm bone mineral content in children. *Acta Paediatr Scand* 1981;70:919–923.
28. Barden HS, Mazess RB, Chesney RW, Rose PG, Chun R. Bone status of children receiving anticonvulsant therapy. *Metab Bone Dis Related Res* 1982;4:43–47.
29. Bettinelli A, Bianchi ML, Aimini E, Ortolani S, Soldati L, Edefonti A. Effects of 1,25-dihydroxy-vitamin-D₃, treatment on mineral balance in children with end stage renal disease undergoing chronic hemofiltration. *Pediatr Res* 1986;20:5–8.

30. Chesney RW, Hamstra AJ, DeLuca HF. Rickets of prematurity: supranormal levels of serum 1,25-dihydroxyvitamin D. *Am J Dis Child* 1981;135:34–37.

31. Chesney RW, Mazess RB, Rose P, Hamstra AJ, DeLuca HF, Breed AL. Long-term influence of calcitriol (1,25-dihydroxyvitamin D) and supplemental phosphate in X-linked hypophosphatemic rickets. *Pediatrics* 1983;71:559–567.

32. Mischler EH, Chesney PJ, Chesney RW, Mazess RB, Rose P. Demineralization in cystic fibrosis detected by direct photon absorptiometry. *Am J Dis Child* 1977;133:632–635.

33. Rosenbloom AL, Lezotte DC, Weber FT, et al. Diminution of bone mass in childhood diabetes. *Diabetica* 1977;26:1052–1055.

34. Shore RM, Chesney RW, Mazess RW, Rose PG, Bargman GJ. Osteopenia in juvenile diabetes. *Calcif Tissue Int* 1981;33:455–457.

35. Shore RM, Chesney RW, Mazess RB, Rose PG, Bargman GJ. Bone mineral status in growth hormone deficiency. *J Pediatr* 1980;96:393–397.

36. Cameron JR, Sorenson J. Measurement of bone mineral in vivo: an improved method. *Science* 1963,142:230–232.

37. Schlenker RA, Von Seggen WW. The distribution of cortical and trabecular bone mass along the lengths of the radius and ulna and the implications for in vivo bone mass measurements. *Calcif Tissue Res* 1976;20:41–52.

38. Mazess RB. Computers used for single and dual photon absorptiometry. In: Gelfand MJ, Thomas SR, eds. *Effective use of computers in nuclear medicine.* New York: McGraw Hill, 1988;503–519.

39. Christiansen C, Rodbro P. Long-term reproducibility of bone mineral content measurements. *Scand J Clin Lab Invest* 1977;37:321–323.

40. Greer FR, McCormick A. Bone growth with low bone mineral content in very low birth weight premature infants. *Pediatr Res* 1986;20:925–928.

41. Greer FR. Determination of radial bone mineral content in low birth weight infants by photon absorptiometry. *J Pediatr* 1988;113:213–219.

42. Mimouni F, Tsang RC. Bone mineral content: data analysis. *J Pediatr* 1988;113:178–180.

43. Steichen JJ, Asch PA, Tsang RC. Bone mineral content measurement in small infants by single-photon absorptiometry: current methodologic issues. *J Pediatr* 1988;113:181–187.

44. Vyhmeister NR, Linkhart TA. Measurement of humerus and radius bone mineral content in the term and preterm infant. *J Pediatr* 1988;113:188–195.

45. Chan G, Leeper L, Book L. Effects of soy formulas on mineral metabolism in term infants. *Am J Dis Child* 1987;141:527–530.

46. Steichen J, Tsang R. Bone mineralization and growth in term infants fed soy-based or cow milk-based formula. *J Pediatr* 1987;110:687–692.

47. Bainbridge RR, Mimouni F, Tsang RC. Bone mineral content of infants fed soy-based formula. *J Pediatr* 1988;113:205–207.

48. Hillman LS. Bone mineral content in term infants fed human milk, cow milk-based formula, or soy-based formula. *J Pediatr* 1988;113:208–212.

49. Chan GM, Mileur L, Hansen JW. Effects of increased calcium and phosphorus formulas and human milk on bone mineralization in preterm infants. *J Pediatr Gastroenterol Nutr* 1986;5:444–449.

50. Venkataraman PS, Blick KE. Effect of mineral supplementation of human milk on bone mineral content and trace element metabolism. *J Pediatr* 1988;113:220–224.

51. Chan GM, Mileur L, Hansen JW. Calcium and phosphorus requirements in bone mineralization of preterm infants. *J Pediatr* 1988;113:225–229.

52. Steichen JJ, Kaplan B, Edwards N, Tsang RC. Bone mineral content in full term infants measured by direct photon absorptiometry. *AJR* 1976;126:1283–1285.

53. Chesney RW, Mehls O, Anast CS, et al. Renal osteodystrophy in children: the role of vitamin D, phosphorus, and parathyroid hormone. *Am J Kidney Dis* 1986;7:275–284.

54. Chesney RW. Metabolic bone disease. *Pediatr Rev* 1984;5:227–237.

55. Chesney RW, Rose PG, Mazess RB. Persistence of diminished bone mineral content following renal transplantation in childhood. *Pediatrics* 1984;73:459–466.

56. Chesney RW, Rose P, Mazess RB, DeLuca HF. Long-term follow-up of bone mineral status of children with renal disease. *Pediatr Nephrol* 1988;2:22–26.

57. Chesney RW, Mazess RB, Rose P. Single photon absorptiometry and dual photon absorptiometry in children. In: Genant HK, ed. *Osteoporosis update.* California: Radiology Research and Education Foundation, 1987;241–246.

58. Shore RM, Chesney RW, Mazess RB, Rose PG, Bargman GJ. Skeletal demineralization in Turner's syndrome. *Calcif Tissue Int* 1982;34:519–522.

59. Arisaka O, Arisaka M, Hosaka A, Shimura N, Yabuta K, Kawaguchi Y. Increase in bone density during testosterone therapy in adolescent hypogonadism [letter]. *Eur J Pediatr* 1989;148:579.
60. Biller BMK, Saxe V, Herzog DB, Rosenthal DI, Holzman S, Klibanski A. Mechanisms of osteoporosis in adult and adolescent women with anorexia nervosa. *J Clin Endocrinol Metab* 1989;68:548–554.
61. Block JE, Piel CF, Selvidge R, Genant HK. Familial hypophosphatemic rickets: bone mass measurements in children following therapy with calcitriol and supplemental phosphate. *Calcif Tissue Int* 1989;44:86–92.
62. Judy PF. A dichromatic attenuation technique for in vivo determination of bone mineral content [Dissertation]. Madison, Wisconsin: University of Wisconsin, Madison, 1971.
63. LeBlanc AD, Evans HJ, March C, Schneider V, Johnson PC, Jhingran SG. Precision of dual photon absorptiometry measurements. *J Nucl Med* 1986;27:1362–1365.
64. Roos BO. Dual photon absorptiometry in lumbar vertebrae. II. Precision and reproducibility. *Acta Radiol* 1975;14:291–303.
65. Schaadt O, Bohr H. Bone mineral by dual-photon absorptiometry: accuracy-precision-sites of measurement. In: Dequekei J, Johnston CC, eds. *Non-invasive bone measurements: methodological problems.* Oxford, England: IRL Press, 1981:59–72.
66. Ythier C, Marchandise X. A method for studying the bone mass: dual-photon absorptiometry. *Pediatrics* 1988;43:371–377.
67. Timperlake RW, Cook SD, Thomas KA, et al. Effects of anticonvulsant drug therapy on bone mineral density in a pediatric population. *J Pediatr Orthop* 1988;8:467–470.
68. Mazess RB, Peppler WW, Chesney RW, Lange TA, Lindgren U, Smith E Jr. Does bone measurement on the radius indicate skeletal status? *J Nucl Med* 1984a;25:281–288.
69. Mazess RB, Peppler WW, Chesney RW, Lange TA, Lindgren U, Smith E Jr. Total body and regional bone mineral by dual-photon absorptiometry in metabolic bone disease. *Calcif Tissue Int* 1984a;36:8–13.
70. Mazess RB, Barden HS, Ohlrich ER. Skeletal and body composition effects of anorexia nervosa. In: *Proceedings of the International Symposium on In Vivo Body Composition Studies [In press].*
71. DeSchepper J, Van den Brock M, De Boeck H, Dirlde MF, Piensz A, Jonckheer MH. Bone mineral measurements by photon absorptiometry: methodologic problems. In: Dequeker J, Geuseno P, Wahner HW, eds. *Determination of lumbar spine bone mineral results by dual photon absorptiometry in children: first results.* Leuven: Leuven University Press, 1988;60–63.
72. Gilsanz V. Quantitative computed tomography in children. In: Genant HK, ed. *Osteoporosis update 1987.* California: Radiology Research and Education Foundation, 1987;181–185.
73. Gilsanz V, Varterasian M, Senac MO Jr, Cann CE. Quantitative spinal mineral analysis in children. *Am Radiol* 1986;29:380–382.
74. Gilsanz V, Carlson ME, Roe TF, Ontega JA. Osteoporosis after cranial irradiation for acute lymphoblastic leukemia. *J Pediatr* 1990;117:238–244.
75. Gibbens DT, Gilsanz V, Boechat MI, Dufer D, Carlson ME, Wang C-I. Osteoporosis in cystic fibrosis. *J Pediatr* 1988;113:295–300.
76. Pacifici R, Rupich R, Griffin M, Chines A, Susman N, Avioli LV. Dual energy radiography versus quantitative computer tomography for the diagnosis of osteoporosis. *J Clin Endocrinol Metab* 1990;70:705–710.
77. Mazess RB. Bone densitometry and monitoring. In: DeLuca HF, Mazess R, eds. *Osteoporosis: physiologic basis, assessment and treatment.* Amsterdam: Elsevier Science Publishing, 1990;63–85.
78. Glastre C, Braillon P, David L, Cochat P, Meunier PJ, Delmas PD. Measurement of bone mineral content of the lumbar spine by dual energy x-ray absorptiometry in normal children: correlations with growth parameters. *J Clin Endocrinol Metab* 1990;70:1330–1333.
79. Poll V, Cooper C, Cawley MID. Broadband ultrasonic attenuation in the os calcis and single photon absorptiometry in the distal forearm: a comparative study. *Clin Phys Physiol Meas* 1986;7:375–379.
80. Wright LL, Glade MJ, Gopal J. The use of transmission ultrasonics to assess bone status in the human newborn. *Pediatr Res* 1987;22:541–544.
81. Koo WK, Tsang R. Bone mineralization in infants. *Prog Food Nutr Sci* 1984;8:229–302.
82. Schanler RJ, Garza C, Nichols BL. Fortified mothers' milk for very low birth weight infants: results of growth and nutrient balance studies. *J Pediatr* 1985;107:437–445.
83. Neville MC, Keller RP, Seacat J, et al. Studies on human lactation. 1. Within-feed and between-breast variation in selected components of human milk. *Am J Clin Nutr* 1984;40:635–646.

84. Karra MV, Udipi SA, Kirksley A, et al. Changes in specific nutrients in breast milk during extended lactation. *Am J Clin Nutr* 1986;40:635–646.
85. Fransson GB, Lonnerdal B. Iron, copper, zinc, calcium and magnesium in human milk fat. *Am J Clin Nutr* 1984;39:185–189.
86. Greer FR, McCormick A, Loker J. Changes in fat concentration of human milk during delivery by intermittent bolus and continuous mechanical pump infusion. *J Pediatr* 1984;105:745–749.
87. Greer FR, Tsang RC, Levin RS, Searcy JE, Wu R, Steichen JJ. Increasing serum calcium and magnesium concentrations in breast-fed infants: longitudinal studies of minerals in human milk and sera of nursing mothers and their infants. *J Pediatr* 1982;100:59–64.
88. Gil A, Sanchez-Medina F. Acid soluble nucleotides of cow's, goat's and sheep's milk at different states of lactation. *J Dairy Res* 1981;48:35–44.
89. Specker BL, Tsang RC, Ho ML, Landi TM, Gratton TL. Low serum calcium and high PTH in infants fed "humanized" cow milk based formula. *Am J Dis Child* (*In press*).
90. Evans JR, Allen AC, Stinson DA, et al. Effect of high-dose vitamin D supplementation on radiographically detectable bone disease of very low birth weight infants. *J Pediatr* 1989;115:779–786.
91. Shenai JP, Reynolds JW, Babson SG. Nutritional balance studies in very-low-birthweight infants: enhanced nutrition retention rates by an experimental formula. *Pediatrics* 1980;66:233–238.
92. Treiber FA, Leonard SB, G Frank, et al. Dietary assessment instruments for preschool children: reliability of parental responses to the 24-hour recall and a food frequency questionnaire. *J Am Diet Assoc* 1990;90:814–820.
93. Klesges RC, Klesges LM, Brown G, Frank GC. Validation of the 24-hour dietary recall in preschool children. *J Am Diet Assoc* 1987;87:1383–1387.
94. Larkin FA, Metzner HL, Thompson FE, Flegal KM, Guire KE. Comparison of estimated nutrient intakes by food frequency and dietary records in adults. *J Am Diet Assoc* 1989;89:215–223.
95. Eck LH, Klesges RC, Hanson CL. Recall of a child's intake from one meal: are parents accurate? *J Am Diet Assoc* 1989;89:784–789.
96. Van Horn LV, Gernhofer N, Moag-Stahlberg A, et al. Dietary assessment in children using electronic methods: telephones and tape recorders. *J Am Diet Assoc* 1990;90:412–416.
97. Krall EA, Dwyer JT. Validity of a food frequency questionnaire and a food diary in a short-term recall situation. *J Am Diet Assoc* 1987;87:1374–1377.
98. Suitor CJW, Gardner J, Willett WC. A comparison of food frequency and diet recall methods in studies of nutrient intake of low-income pregnant women. *J Am Diet Assoc* 1989;89:1786–1794.
99. *Composition of foods: beverages—raw, processed, prepared.* Rev USDA Agriculture Handbook no. 8-14, 1986. Washington, DC: US Government Printing Office.
100. Avioli LV. Intestinal absorption of calcium. *Arch Intern Med* 1972;129:345–355.
101. Bijvoet OLM. Kidney function in calcium and phosphate metabolism. In: Avioli LV, Krane SM, eds. *Metabolic bone disease I.* New York: Academic Press, 1977,50–142.
102. Miller LA, Stapleton FB. Urinary flow rates in children with urolithiasis. *J Urol* 1989;141:918–920.

Calcium Nutriture for Mothers and Children, edited by
Reginald C. Tsang and Francis Mimouni. Carnation
Nutrition Education Series, Vol. 3. Carnation Co.,
Glendale/Raven Press, Ltd., New York © 1992.

The Relation of Calcium Nutrition and Metabolism to Preeclampsia and Premature Labor

Leslie Myatt

*Perinatal Research Institute, Departments of Obstetrics and Gynecology, Pediatrics,
and Physiology and Biophysics, University of Cincinnati College of Medicine,
Cincinnati, Ohio 45267-0526*

Hypertension during pregnancy remains a major problem in perinatology. It may affect up to 10 percent of the 4 million pregnancies in the United States each year (1) and is among the largest causes of maternal morbidity and mortality. Hypertension may develop as a consequence of pregnancy and regress postpartum and is commonly termed pregnancy-induced hypertension (PIH). If underlying hypertension is aggravated by pregnancy, this may be called superimposed PIH. The clinical definition of PIH is a blood pressure of at least 140 mmHg systolic and 90 mmHg diastolic, or an increase in systolic blood pressure of at least 30 mmHg, or an increase in diastolic blood pressure of at least 15 mmHg occurring after the 20th week of gestation and measured on two occasions at least 6 hours apart. In contrast, the well-defined syndrome of preeclampsia is the development of PIH with proteinuria, generalized edema, or both. Although the terms PIH and preeclampsia are often used interchangeably clinically, there is a growing consensus that the presence of proteinuria and/or edema together with PIH is necessary to define clearly those patients with this disease entity as distinct from hypertension from an unknown cause. Preterm labor (after 20 weeks, but before 37 weeks' gestation), which affects up to 9 percent of all pregnancies, is the major single cause of admission to neonatal intensive care units, and is responsible for two-thirds of the 39,000 infant deaths that occur each year in the United States. The societal and economic costs of these disorders are therefore huge. Despite many attempts to identify the etiology of PIH and preeclampsia and of idiopathic preterm labor, the causative and mechanistic factors largely remain unknown. The calcium ion may be a final common effector in both, since increases in intracellular calcium can mediate increased vascular and uterine smooth muscle contractility.

CALCIUM HOMEOSTASIS IN PREGNANCY

Pregnancy *per se* constitutes a major challenge for maternal calcium homeostasis given the dramatic cardiovascular adaptations of pregnancy, the developmental calcium requirements of the fetus, and the ongoing maternal calcium requirement together with the preparation for the subsequent calcium demands of lactation. By term it has been calculated that the fetus accumulates 350 mg calcium/day, the total fetal content at term being 30 g (2). Most of this accretion (80 percent) occurs during the third trimester, the time when PIH or preeclampsia becomes clinically manifest. The current RDA for calcium in pregnancy in the USA is 1,200 mg/day, which is possibly less than that required and in all probability is not reached in a large number of cases. Indeed, in a recent British study, mean intakes of less than 1,000 mg per day were recorded in pregnant women (3). Data on calcium intake in the United States in 1959 (4) showed that adolescent nonpregnant females had average intakes of 1,000 mg/day, which was sufficient to keep them in calcium balance, with a retention of 400 mg/day being needed in the 10–17 year age group for their own mineralization. If the fetal demands of pregnancy are then placed upon this, the positive balance of calcium from a 1 g/day intake will be insufficient (5), and an intake of 2 g/day has been suggested.

To maintain calcium homeostasis during pregnancy, fractional intestinal absorption increases from 27 percent to as high as 50 percent (6) to accommodate the increased requirement. Maternal bone calcium content appears to be preserved during pregnancy but with little data available on bone turnover rates. However, urinary calcium excretion increases during pregnancy (7) due to the increased renal blood flow and glomerular filtration rate. This increase in urinary calcium output occurs even though a positive calcium balance necessary to meet the fetal demands is not achieved. Despite these apparent deficits in calcium intake and balance, normal pregnancies occur; therefore, adaptations in absorption or bone demineralization may be occurring to accommodate the fetal demand and high urinary output. Pregnancy may be associated with "physiologic hyperparathyroidism," which would stimulate bone resorption (8), perhaps as a compensatory response to maintain calcium homeostasis during the vascular adaptation and fetal demands of pregnancy or, alternatively, due to deficient intake. However, recently this view has been challenged with both no change or decreases in parathyroid hormone (PTH) being reported (see the chapter by Pitkin). Bone densitometric measurements have demonstrated no skeletal loss in pregnancy, perhaps because calcitonin response is enhanced to protect the maternal skeleton. The increase in serum PTH concentration output might be a factor responsible for the increase in serum 1,25-dihydroxyvitamin D [1,25(OH)$_2$D] concentrations, which acts to increase intestinal absorption of calcium.

CALCIUM INTAKE AND HYPERTENSION

The concept of a link between calcium intake and the incidence of preeclampsia/eclampsia is not new and has been with us since the 1930s (9).

In nonpregnant subjects, epidemiological studies have shown that restricted dietary calcium is associated with increased blood pressure (10,11). Conversely, a high dietary calcium intake in pregnancy is associated with a relatively low incidence of eclampsia. In countries such as Ethiopia and in rural Guatemala, which have low socioeconomic status and diets poor in proteins and calories, such that a high incidence of eclampsia might be expected, the incidence of eclampsia is in fact low. This is perhaps due to the high dietary intake of calcium (1,075 and 1,100 mg/day) deriving from the staple diet of teff (a grain rich in calcium) and tortillas (made with lime water) in these two countries, respectively (12). This compares with dietary intakes of 240–350 mg calcium/day reported in countries such as Colombia, Thailand, Jamaica, and India, which have a high incidence of preeclampsia (12) and 673 mg/day reported in a low-income U.S. population (13).

Studies with animal models of hypertension have confirmed that restricted dietary calcium is associated with hypertension in nonpregnant (14,15) and pregnant states (16) and that increasing dietary calcium lowers blood pressure (17,18). Recent studies in our institution in twin pregnant sheep (19,20) have shown that either acute starvation or feeding of a low-calcium diet (0.21 percent vs. 0.71 percent) in the third trimester of pregnancy resulted in decreased serum calcium concentrations, increased systemic blood pressure, decreased uteroplacental blood flow, and increased urine protein concentrations. This clinical presentation mimics that of preeclampsia in humans. Infusion of calcium gluconate was sufficient to return serum calcium concentrations to normal in these animals and was accompanied by a reduction in systemic blood pressure and an increase in uterine blood flow. This model of induction of hypertension only produces hypocalcemia in 50 percent of sheep with twin pregnancies, and is not effective in those animals with singleton pregnancies. Whether this differential response represents inherent differences in absorption or retention of calcium or mobilization from skeletal stores remains to be established, but may be a clue to the role of calcium in the development of preeclampsia in humans. Interestingly, reduction of serum ionized calcium and increased blood pressure was associated with preterm labor and delivery in these animals, suggesting that both vascular and uterine smooth muscle reactivity are altered.

CALCIUM SUPPLEMENTATION AND BLOOD PRESSURE

Subsequent to the epidemiological data linking reduced dietary intake of calcium to hypertension, biochemical determinations demonstrated the tendency for individuals with essential hypertension to have low serum ionized calcium concentrations (21,22). These findings have led to dietary calcium supplementation trials in normotensive or hypertensive populations. However, these have yielded variable results. Calcium supplementation has been shown to reduce blood pressure in young adults (23). In a double-blind placebo-controlled trial supplementation of 1,300 mg/day for 12 weeks in normotensive males, mean arterial pressure was modestly but significantly lowered compared with the placebo group (24). In the supplemented group, those patients who responded (≥5 mmHg decrease in mean arterial blood pressure) were older and had a higher mean arterial pressure, higher serum PTH, and lower serum total calcium than did nonresponders (<5 mmHg decrease in blood pressure). Similarly, Grobbee and Hofman (25) and Resnick et al. (26) found antihypertensive effects of calcium in subgroups of hypertensive patients who had elevated PTH concentrations and low serum ionized calcium concentrations. More recently, Luft et al. (27) reported that salt restriction or calcium supplementation (1.5 g/day) decreased blood pressure (2–4 mmHg) in normotensive individuals, whereas potassium supplementation did not. However, the changes in blood pressure with calcium were heterogeneous. In summary, these findings do not suggest a simplistic relationship between calcium supplementation and reduction in blood pressure but that a variety of factors may determine response to this treatment.

CALCIUM METABOLISM IN HYPERTENSIVE PREGNANCY

The biochemical data on mineral metabolism in hypertensive pregnancies are often conflicting and in many cases reflect the inadequacy of study design and inappropriate control groups. In pregnant patients with essential hypertension, significant decreases in serum immunoreactive PTH and ionized calcium, together with an increase in phosphorus, were found compared with nonhypertensive pregnant patients (28). These differences may perhaps have been due to the underlying hypertension prior to pregnancy. In contrast, Richards et al. (29) reported no differences in serum ionized or total calcium among normotensive, chronic hypertensive, mild to moderate pregnancy-induced hypertensive, or severe pregnancy-induced hypertensive/eclamptic pregnant patients. However, these patients were not matched for age. In a black population of severe pregnancy-induced hypertensive/eclamptic patients, total serum calcium concentrations were significantly lower than in normotensive controls, and calculated ionized calcium was significantly reduced in the eclamptic group compared with normotensive and severely hypertensive patients (30). In a recent study (31), we found that, at term, in pregnant patients with pregnancy-induced hypertension serum total and ionized calcium concentrations were significantly lower than in normotensive controls matched for maternal age and gestational age, with the reduction being most marked in those patients with proteinuria. Interestingly, cord blood calcium was also lower in infants of the hypertensive patients, although not significantly lower than controls. These findings are in agreement with the reduced cord blood ionized calcium found in infants of essential hypertensive mothers compared with those of normotensive mothers (28).

Normotensive pregnancy is associated with increased urinary calcium excretion (7). Hypocalciuria has, however, been reported in pregnancy-induced hypertension/preeclampsia. In the study of Pederson et al. (32), reduced fractional urinary excretion of calcium was seen in the third trimester in hypertensive patients compared with controls despite the fact that no differences in total serum calcium concentrations were found between the two groups of patients. Taufield et al. (33) confirmed the hypocalciuria in preeclamptic patients or hypertensive patients with superimposed preeclampsia, suggesting that it was due to either reduced glomerular filtration rate or increased tubular reabsorption compared to the normotensive state. The hypocalciuria was not found in pregnant women with transient or chronic hypertension. Whether hypocalciuria is a specific feature of preeclampsia or a nonspecific manifestation of renal insufficiency found in preeclampsia is unclear (34). However, screening for a low calcium/creatinine ratio in the late second/early third trimester of pregnancy has been suggested as a useful test in predicting the subsequent development of preeclampsia (35), but it needs further verification.

INTRACELLULAR CALCIUM IN HYPERTENSION

The mechanistic linkage between reduced dietary intake of calcium and the consequent reduced serum calcium concentrations to the development of increased vascular smooth muscle tone is largely ill defined. The calcium ion appears to be the final common mediator of smooth muscle contractility. Increased intracellular calcium causes contraction, and there is growing evidence that hypertension is associated with increased intracellular calcium concentration. Measurements of intracellular calcium in blood cells are being used as a proxy for measurement of smooth muscle intracellular calcium in hypertensive individuals. In nonpregnant, black, hypertensive patients, platelet membrane-bound calcium concentration was found to be significantly higher compared with normotensive controls by measurement with a fluorescent indicator (36). Similarly, in essential hypertensive subjects, platelet intracellular calcium concentration (measured with the fluorescent indicators quin-2 and fura-2) was significantly higher than in normotensive controls and significantly correlated with systolic blood pressure (37). However, lymphocyte intracellular calcium did not correlate with blood pressure, in agreement with other reports (38). Therefore, differences in calcium handling in hypertension only appear to be expressed in certain cell types.

Similar studies have been performed in preeclampsia. Erythrocyte intracellular calcium was significantly increased in patients with pregnancy-induced hypertension compared with gestational age-matched (≤ 35 weeks) normotensive controls (39), whereas intracellular sodium, potassium, and magnesium concentrations were not different. In contrast, Barr et al. (40) found no differences in basal or adenosine diphosphate (ADP)-stimulated platelet intracellular calcium concentrations between nonpregnant patients and those in the third trimester of pregnancy who were either normotensive or had pregnancy-induced hypertension or preeclampsia. There was, however, a tendency for a reduction in response of platelet calcium concentration to 5-hydroxytryptamine stimulation, which was most marked in preeclampsia. However, Kilby et al. (41) reported significantly increased platelet intracellular calcium in proteinuric, hypertensive, pregnant primigravidae and a significant correlation between platelet intracellular calcium and systolic blood pressure. Recently, in a prospective study of platelet intracellular calcium throughout the three trimesters of pregnancy in young black patients, Zemel et al. (42) reported that, whereas there was no difference in basal platelet intracellular calcium at any time, those patients who subsequently developed preeclampsia had an exaggerated increase in intracellular calcium in response to stimulation by arginine vasopressin (AVP). This response was maintained in the second and third trimesters and was a sensitive predictor of preeclampsia. Unfortunately, the authors did not report whether the exaggerated response to AVP was present in the nonpregnant state. Overall, there is still discordance relating to intracellular calcium concentrations in hypertensive pregnancy, perhaps due to differences in techniques, patient populations, or cell types studied.

DIETARY CALCIUM SUPPLEMENTATION IN PREGNANCY

The relationship of overall nutrition to outcome in pregnancy (including eclampsia and preterm labor) has long been recognized (43), and early dietary supplementation studies involved supplementation with a series of nutrients that included calcium. The result of these trials was a reduction in the incidence of eclampsia, yet with no clear knowledge of the component of the supplement responsible. Osofsky (13) supplemented a lower income pregnant population with a protein/mineral supplement (Meritene) and found significantly less of an increase in systolic and diastolic blood pressures in supplemented versus non-supplemented patients. The mean daily calcium intake in the supplemented group was 1,028 mg compared with 673 mg in the nonsupplemented.

A natural consequence of the epidemiological and biochemical data supporting a role for reduced calcium intake in the genesis of hypertension, and the nutrient supplementation studies, has been trials of dietary supplementation with calcium. As previously stated, the dietary supplementation data from nonpregnant populations have been equivocal. However, it is perhaps to be expected that results may be more definitive in pregnant individuals, in whom the challenges to calcium homeostasis and the necessary intake are greater. In two separate but complementary studies (44,45), Belizan, Villar, and coworkers studied the effect of dietary calcium supplementation on blood pressure during pregnancy and on clinical outcome. In their earlier study (44), 36 urban Guatemalan women with singleton pregnancies were randomized to receive 1 g/day or 2 g/day calcium, or placebo from 15 weeks' gestation until term. Whereas both the calcium-supplemented groups had significantly lower diastolic blood pressures between 20 and 24 weeks' gestation compared with placebo, only the patients receiving 2 g calcium/day had significantly lower blood pressures in the third trimester. No differences were observed in blood total calcium, magnesium, phosphorus, or protein concentrations among the three groups in this population, who had a usual dietary intake of calcium of 700 mg/day. In a later study combining 34 black patients from John Hopkins Hospital, Baltimore, and 18 white patients from Rosario, Argentina, a double-blind, randomized, placebo-controlled trial of supplementation with 1.5 g/day calcium after the 26th week of gestation was performed (45). After adjustment for race and initial blood pressure, subjects in the calcium-supplemented group had significantly lower systolic and diastolic blood pressures at term compared with the placebo group and a lower (4.0 percent vs. 11.1

percent, N.S.) incidence of pregnancy-induced hypertension. Assuming a normal distribution of blood pressure, the reduction in diastolic blood pressure (from 76.99 mmHg to 72.05 mmHg) found in this study with calcium supplementation would reduce the incidence of PIH from 10 percent to 4 percent. By comparing their two studies, the authors also claimed a dose-dependent effect of calcium supplementation in reducing blood pressure in pregnancy.

Interestingly, an earlier placebo-controlled study in India of 375 mg/day calcium and 1,200 IU/day vitamin D supplementation from 20 to 24 weeks' gestation to term significantly reduced systolic and diastolic blood pressure by 36 weeks' gestation but only produced a slight nonsignificant reduction in the incidence of toxemia (46). In another study involving Japanese women, Kawasaki et al. (47) found supplementation with a lower amount of calcium (600 mg/day of calcium aspartate = 156 g/day elemental calcium) from 22 weeks to term to blunt vascular reactivity to infused angiotensin II. There was no alteration in blood calcium measurements nor reduction in blood pressure. Exaggerated vascular reactivity to infused angiotensin II is purportedly characteristic of PIH and is used as a screening test for development of PIH (48). The mechanism whereby calcium supplementation reduces response to angiotensin II and yet does not affect blood pressure is unclear. In this light, it is interesting that in the hypocalcemic sheep model pressor responses to angiotensin II and norepinephrine were significantly reduced in animals on a low-calcium diet. Furthermore, the blood pressure response to infusion of these agonists was positively correlated with blood ionized calcium concentrations (49).

Lopez-Jaramillo et al. (50) performed a double-blind randomized placebo-controlled trial of 2 g/day elemental calcium supplementation from 24 weeks' gestation until term in a population of 106 nulliparous women in Quito, Ecuador. These women had a usual dietary intake of calcium of 300 mg/day (51). The supplementation was associated with a significantly decreased risk of PIH (4.1 percent in the treatment group vs. 27.9 percent in the placebo group) and also resulted in significant reductions in systolic and diastolic blood pressure over the duration of treatment. A significantly greater rate of increase in blood pressure throughout gestation was found in the placebo group. Serum ionized calcium concentrations were significantly higher in the supplemented group compared with placebo and were increased by week 28 of gestation to a concentration seen in the nonpregnant postpartum period and remained at this level throughout the rest of gestation. In contrast, serum ionized calcium in the placebo group fell further, from 24 weeks' gestation to 32 weeks' gestation. It remained low until delivery, when the concentration increased again in the postpartum period and was not significantly different from that in the supplemental group. Thus, in the placebo group of this population with poor dietary calcium intake, there was a progressive decline in serum ionized calcium throughout gestation presumably related to fetal demands. Calcium supplementation appears to be able to prevent this decline and maintain ionized calcium concentrations at the nonpregnant level. Birth weight was slightly, but not significantly, higher (3,097 g vs. 2,832 g) in the supplemented group, to some extent probably due to the significantly increased duration of gestation (39.3 weeks vs. 38.7 weeks).

A similar trial but with a different outcome was performed in a predominantly (94 percent) black, adolescent population in Baltimore (52). Patients (17 years of age or less, n = 189) were randomized to receive either 2 g/day of elemental calcium supplementation or placebo in a double-blind, randomized trial from 24 weeks' gestation until term. Normal dietary intake of calcium in these patients was 1,200 mg/day. The calcium-supplemented group had a significantly lower incidence of preterm delivery (<37 weeks, 7.4 percent vs. 21.1 percent), spontaneous labor and preterm delivery (6.4 percent vs. 17.9 percent), and low birth weight (9.6 percent vs. 21.1 percent). Life table analysis showed a shift to a greater gestational age at delivery in the calcium group (39.2 weeks) compared with the placebo group (37.9 weeks), which was probably responsible for the increased mean birth weight of the calcium group (3,128 g vs. 2,939 g). Interestingly, however, there was no significant reduction in the incidence of either PIH or preeclampsia, although the rates were lower in the calcium group. This finding may reflect the low incidence of PIH and preeclampsia in this population, which attends a well-organized adolescent pregnancy clinic, or the fact that their basal calcium intake was higher than in the Ecuadorian studies.

The disparate results obtained among the clinical trials performed to date make it difficult to draw firm conclusions regarding the effect of dietary calcium supplementation in pregnancy. What they do show is that the dietary, environmental, social, and genetic factors particular to each patient population may be important determinants of response. It is, however, tempting to speculate that supplementation with up to 2 g elemental calcium/day may decrease reactivity of smooth muscle of vascular or uterine origin, the net result being reduced blood pressure or reduced uterine contractility. It is still unclear whether the calcium supplementation may be correcting a deficiency of dietary and blood calcium, as suggested by the study of Lopez-Jaramillo et al. (50), or is a pharmacologic effect in patients with dietary calcium intakes in pregnancy close to the RDA (52).

BIOCHEMICAL MECHANISMS

The biochemical mechanisms that underlie the apparent paradox of decreased extracellular calcium but increased intracellular calcium in hypertension are unclear at present. Attention has primarily focused on the action of PTH on cation transport at the cell membrane and the activity of the transporters themselves (Fig. 1). A reduction in the activity of Na^+/K^+ adenosinetriphosphatase (ATPase) and a relative increase in the activity of Ca^{2+} ATPase has been reported in erythrocyte membranes of gestational hypertensive women compared with normotensive pregnant women (53). The increase in Ca^{2+} ATPase may be a compensatory response as the cell tries to extrude high levels of intracellular free calcium, which, in turn, may arise from decreased sodium–calcium exchange in the presence of high intracellular sodium due to the reduced Na^+/K^+ ATPase (54). PTH is thought to be a calcium ionophore in vascular smooth muscle (55), which would directly increase intracellular calcium, and has also purportedly been shown to inhibit erythrocyte Na^+/K^+ ATPase, which

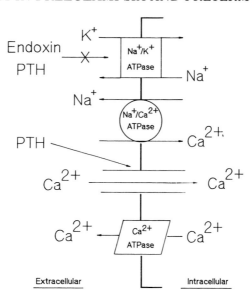

FIG. 1. Mechanisms for maintenance of intracellular calcium homeostasis. ATPase, adenosine-triphophatase; PTH, parathyroid hormone.

would indirectly increase intracellular calcium (39). Interestingly, concentrations of both serum PTH and "endoxin," a natriuretic substance that inhibits Na^+/K^+ ATP-ase, were higher in patients with PIH compared with controls, although the increase was only significant for endoxin (39). In these patients, however, no differences were seen in serum ionized calcium and magnesium concentrations. Decreased calcium intake and/or intestinal absorption or increased urinary output of calcium theoretically could result in increased PTH. Interestingly, in supplementation studies (44–56), patients with the highest level of calcium supplementation (2 g/day) had the lowest serum PTH concentrations at term. In animal studies, Belizan et al. (57) found that rats fed on a calcium-free diet developed increased blood pressure but that parathyroidectomy was able to prevent this increase. The parathyroidectomized calcium-free rats actually had lower blood pressures than control animals fed a normal calcium diet. These data emphasize the role that PTH may play in control of blood pressure.

In addition to the direct effects of calcium on smooth muscle cell contractility, which regulates blood pressure, calcium may also have indirect effects via the regulation of production of other vasoactive agents (Fig. 2). It has been proposed that extracellular calcium may stimulate prostacyclin synthesis from arachidonic acid by vascular tissue, the prostacyclin acting as a vasodilator (58). Alternatively, the concentration of calcium in extracellular medium can regulate the synthesis of the endothelial cell-derived vasodilator agent nitric oxide. Calcium concentrations of 0.5–1.25 mM stimulate nitric oxide synthesis, but with inhibition by 1.25–2 mM calcium

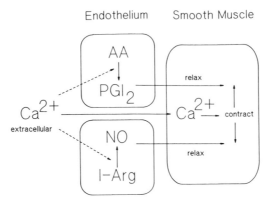

FIG. 2. Direct and indirect actions of calcium on smooth muscle. AA, arachidonic acid; L-Arg, L-arginine; NO, nitric oxide; PGI₂, prostacyclin.

(59). Nitric oxide synthesized from the amino acid L-arginine in endothelium appears to have a physiologic role in the control of vascular tone *in vivo* (60).

CONCLUSIONS

The weight of evidence implying a role for inadequate dietary intake of calcium in the etiology of hypertension in nonpregnant individuals and in PIH and preeclampsia during pregnancy is impressive. It should not, however, be assumed that such deficiency is the primary etiologic factor in these conditions. In particular, the well-described uteroplacental pathology of PIH/preeclampsia (61) involving an inadequate or absent secondary wave of trophoblast invasion of the maternal spiral arteries and the presence of acute atherosis in these vessels, which is suggested to be the common etiologic factor, implies that the role of dietary calcium insufficiency may be as an additional predisposing or compounding risk factor. Furthermore, differences in the capacity of maternal homeostatic mechanisms to reset when faced with the additional fetal calcium demands may also determine the ultimate response. In the absence of measurements of smooth muscle intracellular calcium concentration, the tacit assumption has to be made that these concentrations are increased in PIH/preeclampsia and that such increases are reflected in platelets and erythrocytes. If such increases in intracellular calcium occur in both vascular and uterine smooth muscle, then a common mechanism can be invoked for the development of both hypertension and preterm labor. The mechanisms underlying the beneficial effects claimed in the dietary calcium supplementation studies to date are again difficult to interpret. In populations with inadequate mineral nutrition, supplementation may simply be correcting their deficiency and may thus lead to beneficial outcome. The benefits that are claimed in populations with a dietary calcium intake closer to the RDA are more problematic to explain in physiologic terms. Either there is still a substantial negative calcium balance in some patients at these intakes (particularly perhaps adolescents), which is corrected by supplementation, or, alternatively, supplementation with 2 g calcium/day has a pharmacologic effect opposite to that of deficiency and, hence, reduces intracellular calcium concentrations and vascular reactivity. The biochemical measurements to verify these propositions are missing from the supplementation studies. Furthermore, the potential benefits of dietary calcium supplementation to the pregnant population as a whole must be tested by large-scale longitudinal, randomized, double-blind, placebo-controlled studies.

ACKNOWLEDGMENTS

The assistance of Ms. Beth Bourne and Ms. Joelene Dixon in preparation of this manuscript is gratefully acknowledged.

REFERENCES

1. Pritchard JA, MacDonald PC, Gant NF, eds. Hypertensive disorders in pregnancy. In: *Williams obstetrics,* 18th ed. Norwalk, CT: Appleton-Century-Crofts, 1985:525–560.
2. Forkes GB. Calcium accumulation by the human fetus. *Pediatrics* 1976;57:976–977.
3. Schofield C, Stewart J, Wheeler E. The diets of pregnant and post-pregnant women in different social groups in London and Edinburgh: calcium, iron, retinol, ascorbic acid and folic acid. *Br J Nutr* 1989;62:363–377.
4. Oblson MA, Stearns G. Calcium intake of children and adults. *Fed Proc* 1959;18:1076–1085.
5. Duggin GG, Lyneham RC, Dale NE, Evans RA, Tiller DJ. Calcium balance in pregnancy. *Lancet* 1974;11:926–927.
6. Heaney RP, Skillman TG. Calcium metabolism in normal human pregnancy. *J Clin Endocrinol Metab* 1971;36:661–670.
7. Howarth AT, Morgan DB, Payne RB. Urinary excretion of calcium in late pregnancy and its relation to creatinine clearance. *Am J Obstet Gynecol* 1977;129:499–502.
8. Pitkin RM. Calcium metabolism in pregnancy and the perinatal period: a review. *Am J Obstet Gynecol* 1985;151:99–109.
9. Theobald GW. Calcium and vitamins A and D on incidence of pregnancy-induced toxaemia. *Lancet* 1937;1:1397–1399.
10. McCarron DA, Morris CD, Cole C. Dietary calcium in human hypertension. *Science* 1982;217:267–269.
11. Kesteloot H, Joossens JV. Relationship of dietary sodium, potassium, calcium and magnesium with blood pressure. Belgian Interuniversity Research on Nutrition and Health. *Hypertension* 1988;12:594–599.
12. Belizan JM, Villar J. The relationship between calcium intake and edema proteinuria and hypertension gestosis: an hypothesis. *Am J Clin Nutr* 1980;33:2202–2210.
13. Osofsky HJ. Relationship between prenatal medical and nutritional measures, pregnancy outcome and early infant development in an urban poverty setting. *Am J Obstet Gynecol* 1975;123:682–690.
14. Furspan P, Rinaldi GJ, Hoffman K, Bohr DF. Dietary calcium and cell membrane abnormality in genetic hypertension. *Hypertension* 1989;13:727–730.
15. Hatton DC, Scrogin KE, Metz JA, McCarron DA. Dietary calcium alters blood pressure reactivity in spontaneously hypertensive rats. *Hypertension* 1989;13:622–629.
16. Belizan JM, Pineda O, Sainz E, Meneridez LA, Villar J. Rise of blood pressure in calcium-deprived pregnant rats. *Am J Obstet Gynecol* 1981;141:163–169.
17. Ayachi S. Increased dietary calcium lowers blood pressure in the spontaneously hypertensive rat. *Metabolism* 1979;12:1234–1238.
18. Peuler JD, Morgan DA, Mark AL. High calcium diet reduces blood pressure in Dahl-salt sensitive rats by neural mechanisms. *Hypertension* 1987;9(Suppl III):159–165.

19. Prada J, Ross R, Clark K. Hypertensive effects of starvation: Role of Ca^{2+} in the pregnant sheep. Presented at the 34th Meeting of the Society for Gynecologic Investigation, 1987. Abstract 62P.
20. Prada J, Brockman D, Moore K, Clark K. Hypocalcemia leads to pregnancy-induced hypertension in sheep. Presented at the 35th Meeting of the Society for Gynecologic Investigation, 1988. Abstract 7.
21. McCarron DA. Low serum concentrations of ionized calcium in patients with hypertension. *N Engl J Med* 1982;307:226–228.
22. Resnick LM. Uniformity and diversity of calcium metabolism in hypertension. A conceptual framework. *Am J Med* 1987;82(Suppl IB):16–26.
23. Belizan JM, Villar J, Pineda O, et al. Reduction of blood pressure with calcium supplementation in young adults. *JAMA* 1983;249:1161–1165.
24. Lyle RM, Melby CL, Hyner GC. Metabolic differences between subjects whose blood pressure did or did not respond to oral calcium supplementation. *Am J Clin Nutr* 1988;47:1030–1035.
25. Grobbee DE, Hofman A. Effect of calcium supplementation on diastolic blood pressure in young people with mild hypertension. *Lancet* 1986;II:703–707.
26. Resnick LM, Nicholson JP, Laragh JH. Calcium metabolism in essential hypertension: relationship to altered renin system activity. *Fed Proc* 1986;45:2739–2745.
27. Luft FC, Miller JZ, Lyle R, et al. The effect of dietary interventions to reduce blood pressure in normal humans. *J Am Coll Nutr* 1989;8:495–503.
28. Varner MW, Cruikshank DP, Pitkin RM. Calcium metabolism in the hypertensive mother, fetus and newborn infant. *Am J Obstet Gynecol* 1983;147:762–765.
29. Richards SR, Nelson DM, Zuspan FP. Calcium levels in normal and hypertensive pregnant patients. *Am J Obstet Gynecol* 1984;149:168–171.
30. Moodley J, Rampersadh S, Becker P, Norman RJ, O'Dondl D. Serum calcium ion concentrations in eclampsia. *S Afr Med J* 1987;72:382–385.
31. Waddell BJ, Ross R, Myatt L. Disturbed fetal and maternal calcium and magnesium homeostasis in hypertensive pregnancy. Presented at VII World Congress of Hypertension in Pregnancy, 1990. Abstract p. 269.
32. Pedersen EB, Johannesen P, Kristensen S, et al. Calcium, parathyroid hormone and calcitonin in normal pregnancy and preeclampsia. *Gynecol Obstet Invest* 1984;18:156–164.
33. Taufield PA, Ales KL, Resnick LM, Druzin ML, Gertner JM, Laragh JH. Hypocalciuria in preeclampsia. *N Engl J Med* 1987;316:715–718.
34. Graber ML, Moore B. Hypocalciuria in preeclampsia. *N Engl J Med* 1987;317:897–899.
35. Rodriguez MH, Masaki DI, Mestman J, Kumar D, Rude R. Calcium/creatinine ratio and microalbuminuria in the prediction of preeclampsia. *Am J Obstet Gynecol* 1988;159:1452–1455.
36. Cooper R, Lipowski J, Ford E, Shamsi N, Feinberg H, LeBreton G. Increased membrane-bound calcium in platelets of hypertensive patients. *Hypertension* 1989;13:139–144.
37. Pritchard K, Raine AG, Ashley CC, et al. Correlation of blood pressure in normotensive and hypertensive individuals with platelet but not lymphocyte intracellular free calcium concentrations. *Clin Sci* 1989;76:631–635.
38. Lew PD, Favre L, Waldvogel FA, Vallotton MB. Cytosolic free calcium and intracellular calcium stores in neutrophils from hypertensive subjects. *Clin Sci* 1985;69:227–230.
39. Sowers JR, Zemel MB, Bronsteen RA, et al. Erythrocyte cation metabolism in preeclampsia. *Am J Obstet Gynecol* 1989;161:441–445.
40. Barr SM, Lees KR, Butters L, O'Donnell A, Rubin PC. Platelet intracellular free calcium concentration in normotensive and hypertensive pregnancies in the human. *Clin Sci* 1989;76:67–71.
41. Kilby MD, Broughton-Pipkin F, Heptinstall S, Symonds EM. A comparison of platelet cytosolic free calcium concentrations in both normotensive and hypertensive primigravidae. Presented at VII World Congress of Hypertension in Pregnancy, 1990. Abstract p. 72.
42. Zemel MB, Zemel PC, Berry S, et al. Altered platelet calcium metabolism as an early predictor of increased peripheral vascular resistance and preeclampsia in urban black women. *N Engl J Med* 1990;323:434–438.
43. Tompkins WT, Wiehl DG. Nutritional deficiencies as a causal factor in toxaemia and premature labor. *Am J Obstet Gynecol* 1951;62:898–919.
44. Belizan JM, Villar J, Zalazar A, Rojas J, Chan D, Bryce GF. Preliminary evidence of the effect of calcium supplementation on blood pressure in normal pregnant women. *Am J Obstet Gynecol* 1983;146:175–180.
45. Villar J, Repke J, Belizan JM, Pareja G. Calcium supplementation reduces blood pressure during pregnancy: results of a randomized controlled clinical trial. *Obstet Gynecol* 1987;70:317–322.

46. Marya RK, Rathee S, Manrow M. Effect of calcium and vitamin D supplementation on toxaemia of pregnancy. *Gynecol Obstet Invest* 1987;24:38–42.
47. Kawasaki N, Matsui K, Ito M, et al. Effect of calcium supplementation on the vascular sensitivity to angiotensin II in pregnant women. *Am J Obstet Gynecol* 1985;153:576–582.
48. Gant NF, Daley GL, Chand S, Whalley PJ, MacDonald PC. A study of angiotensin II pressor response throughout primigravid pregnancy. *J Clin Invest* 1973;52:2682–2689.
49. Prada JA, Clark KE. Modulation of pressor responsiveness by circulating levels of Ca^{2+} in twin pregnant ewes. Presented at the 37th Annual Meeting of the Society for Gynecologic Investigation, 1990. Abstract 527.
50. Lopez-Jaramillo P, Narvaez M, Weigel RM, Yepez R. Calcium supplementation reduces the risk of pregnancy-induced hypertension in an Andes population. *Br J Obstet Gynaecol* 1989;96:648–655.
51. Lopez-Jaramillo P, Narvaez M, Yepez R. Effect of calcium supplementation on the vascular sensitivity to angiotensin II in pregnant women. *Am J Obstet Gynecol* 1987;156:261–262.
52. Villar J, Repke J. Calcium supplementation during pregnancy may reduce preterm delivery in high-risk populations. *Am J Obstet Gynecol* 1990;163:1124–1131.
53. Tranquili AL, Rabini RA, Cugini AM, et al. Calcium and sodium transport in gestational hypertension. *Int J Cardiol* 1989;25:S53–S55.
54. Friedman SM. Cellular ionic perturbations in hypertension. *J Hypertens* 1983;1:109–114.
55. Schleiffer R, Berthelot A, Gairard A. Effects of parathyroid extract on blood pressure and arterial contraction and on Ca exchange in isolated aorta in the rat. *Blood Vessels* 1979;16:220–221.
56. Belizan JM, Villar J, Repke J. The relationship between calcium intake and pregnancy-induced hypertension: up-to-date evidence. *Am J Obstet Gynecol* 1988;158:898–902.
57. Belizan JM, Villar J, Self S, Pineda O, Gonzalez I, Sainz E. The mediating role of the parathyroid gland in the effect of low calcium intake on blood pressure in the rat. *Arch Latinoam Nutr* 1984;34:666–675.
58. Lopez-Jaramillo P, Guarner F, Moncada S. Effects of calcium and parathyroid hormone on prostacyclin synthesis by vascular tissue. *Life Sci* 1987;40:983–986.
59. Lopez-Jaramillo P, Gonzalez MC, Palmer RMJ, Moncada S. The crucial role of physiological Ca^{2+} concentrations in the production of endothelial nitric oxide and the control of vascular tone. *Br J Pharmacol* 1990;101:489–493.
60. Rees DD, Palmer RMJ, Moncada S. Role of endothelium-derived nitric oxide in the regulation of blood pressure. *Proc Natl Acad Sci USA* 1989;86:3375–3378.
61. Khong TY, DeWolf F, Robertson WB, Brosens I. Inadequate maternal vascular response to placentation in pregnancies complicated by pre-eclampsia and by small-for-gestational age infants. *Br J Obstet Gynaecol* 1986;93:1049–1059.

Subject Index

143